Low Vision Aids Practice

Low Vision Aids Practice
Third Edition

Ajay Kumar Bhootra
B Optom DOS FAO FOAI FCLI
ICLEP FIACLE (Australia)
Diploma in Sportvision (UK)

Ex-CEO and Dean
Krishnalaya School of Optometry
Kolkata, West Bengal, India

Foreword
Sambuddha Kundu

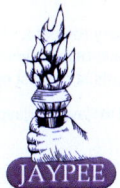

JAYPEE BROTHERS MEDICAL PUBLISHERS
The Health Sciences Publisher
New Delhi | London

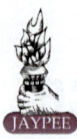 **Jaypee Brothers Medical Publishers (P) Ltd**

Headquarters
Jaypee Brothers Medical Publishers (P) Ltd
EMCA House, 23/23-B
Ansari Road, Daryaganj
New Delhi 110 002, India
Landline: +91-11-23272143, +91-11-23272703
+91-11-23282021, +91-11-23245672
Email: jaypee@jaypeebrothers.com

Corporate Office
Jaypee Brothers Medical Publishers (P) Ltd
4838/24, Ansari Road, Daryaganj
New Delhi 110 002, India
Phone: +91-11-43574357
Fax: +91-11-43574314
Email: jaypee@jaypeebrothers.com

Overseas Office
J.P. Medical Ltd
83 Victoria Street, London
SW1H 0HW (UK)
Phone: +44 20 3170 8910
Fax: +44 (0)20 3008 6180
Email: info@jpmedpub.com

Website: www.jaypeebrothers.com
Website: www.jaypeedigital.com

© 2023, Jaypee Brothers Medical Publishers

The views and opinions expressed in this book are solely those of the original contributor(s)/author(s) and do not necessarily represent those of editor(s) and publisher of the book.

All rights reserved. No part of this publication may be reproduced, stored or transmitted in any form or by any means, electronic, mechanical, photocopying, recording or otherwise, without the prior permission in writing of the publishers.

All brand names and product names used in this book are trade names, service marks, trademarks or registered trademarks of their respective owners. The publisher is not associated with any product or vendor mentioned in this book.

Medical knowledge and practice change constantly. This book is designed to provide accurate, authoritative information about the subject matter in question. However, readers are advised to check the most current information available on procedures included and check information from the manufacturer of each product to be administered, to verify the recommended dose, formula, method and duration of administration, adverse effects and contraindications. It is the responsibility of the practitioner to take all appropriate safety precautions. Neither the publisher nor the author(s)/editor(s) assume any liability for any injury and/or damage to persons or property arising from or related to use of material in this book.

This book is sold on the understanding that the publisher is not engaged in providing professional medical services. If such advice or services are required, the services of a competent medical professional should be sought.

Every effort has been made where necessary to contact holders of copyright to obtain permission to reproduce copyright material. If any have been inadvertently overlooked, the publisher will be pleased to make the necessary arrangements at the first opportunity.

Inquiries for bulk sales may be solicited at: jaypee@jaypeebrothers.com

Low Vision Aids Practice

First Edition: 2005
Second Edition: 2007
Third Edition: **2023**

ISBN: 978-93-5696-107-4

Printed at India

Foreword

I am delighted to write the foreword for the 3rd edition of *Low Vision Aids Practice* by Ajay Kumar Bhootra. I have referred many patients of low vision to Mr Bhootra. He managed all my patients very efficiently and ethically. One day during an informal meeting, he showed me the manuscript of this edition. I was very much impressed by the methodical explanation of specialized low vision tests that he has covered in the book. Other contents were also very relevant and beautifully written. To me the book looked very well organized.

I would personally like to recommend all the students of optometry and also all those practitioners who are working with visually impaired patients in any capacity to read this book. It is a practice-oriented book and is very simply written.

It is my belief that the book will certainly provide an effective learning experience.

Sambuddha Kundu
MBBS (Cal), DOMS
Eye Surgeon and Medical Vitreo Retina Fellow
Aravind Eye Hospital
India

Preface to the Third Edition

When Mrs Samina Khan of Jaypee Publishers Pvt Ltd approached me with an idea of revisiting the 2007 edition of Low Vision Aids Practice, I was excited. The reasons were simple. I also wanted to revise it to make it more elaborate and updated because when I wrote its first edition in 2005, the objective was to create a basic resource material on low vision for practitioners as well as for students and unfortunately in 2007 when the second edition was published, I could not make substantial addition. The past few years have seen lot of developments not only in terms of innovations in the field of visual aids but also in terms of number of practicing optometrists. Several manufacturers have begun manufacturing different types of aids and devices, and many optometrists have started incorporating low vision care into their practice. I have been also able to build up my practice in low vision care and have had the opportunity to see several patients that had enabled me to gain more experience in real life practice. Real life experiences are great source of learning. We get to learn the most from experiences of our own as well as of others. So, I figured it is the time to rewrite this book and make it more elaborate and informative as a resource material, for eye care professionals and students alike.

The new third edition of *Low Vision Aids Practice* is more elaborate and very comprehensive. It contains 16 chapters, each of which has been conceived and designed with specific objectives. Chapters 1 and 2 set the tone to go deeper into the core of the subject. In these two chapters, I synthesizes the basic fundamentals of the subject and presents the human element as can be observed in many low vision patients. Chapters 3 to 5 are about the tests that form the part of preliminary examination procedure needed for low vision patients. Chapter 6 is unique and is probably the most critical for what can probably be said to be the most important factor for building up the successful low vision practice. Chapters 7 and 8 are about the specialized procedures that are usually applied routinely in low vision practice but may not be applied in general eye examination practice. Chapter 9 talks about causes of low vision, whereas Chapters 10,

11, and 12 explain in detail the aids and devices that are commonly prescribed to low vision patients and related optics. Chapters 13 and 14 are very important and talk about the master idea that would transform your practice and make you a creative choreographer of your own success as the low vision practitioner. Chapter 15 talks about allied specialized services that are also important for holistic rehabilitation of visual impaired patients. Even though you are the master of low vision practice, at times you will need to refer your patients to other professional experts. Chapter 16 is the last chapter, although it has nothing to do with tests and procedures, it is very important in terms of the fact that it tries to explain that plans and preparations are very important to build up a successful practice. Any compromise in this area may prove disastrous.

In pursuit of making the book more student-friendly, I have also added multiple choice questions and self-practice questions at the end of each chapter. The students can practice writing answers to the questions given at the end of each chapter and work with multiple choice questions. Despite these enhancements, there is further scope for improvements. The readers may take the help of other textbooks available on the subject to get into more detailing.

However, I am sure it will serve its purpose in more improved manner than before. With this hope, I wish you a good read and the very best in your journey toward becoming a successful low vision practitioner.

Ajay Kumar Bhootra

Preface to the First Edition

Low vision can affect everybody—rich and poor, old and young, all races and ethnic backgrounds equally. Still it is more commonly associated with the older population of our society. There is no doubt that there is an increasing need for eye practitioners, to become more involved in the field of low vision rehabilitation, either by actively participating or becoming more involved in the referral process. It is with this in mind that this book has been written. For those practitioners who would like to become involved in the field of low vision rehabilitation or for those who are presently optometry or ophthalmology students, this book provides the basic and essential informations to begin work in this rewarding field both for the practitioners as well as the patients. I believe that even the practising low vision practitioners will also find the informations in this book helpful.

In conclusion, I would like to write that I have tried to simplify the text of the subject to the maximum possibility. I would be highly satisfied if this book serves the purpose of those for whom this has been written.

Ajay Kumar Bhootra

Acknowledgments

As far as I understand no creation in this world is a solo effort. Neither is this book. I have received enormous inputs of several persons from the time I conceived the idea of this book to its present shape. I would like to acknowledge everybody's effort and would like to thank all of them for bringing it to this shape. Special thanks to:

My readers and students for their support and love

God, who cares for me

My amazing list of patients and clients because of whom I could have so varied experience.

All my trainers and coaches who had been instrumental in providing me training on different occasions.

My friends and family members

And all the people I met during my working experience and trainings who helped me understand my subject.

Above all, all the members of my organization Himalaya Optical.

I am fond of reading books on various subjects. That is why while reading this book you may notice that the contents of this book are influenced by several books. Probably, that makes the disc roll in favor of the book.

And finally, I would like to re-collect my old memories when I had my mentor Late Sri KK Binani who taught me, encouraged me, and believed in me.

Contents

1. **Low Vision** 1
   - Clinical Characteristics of Low Vision 3
   - Psychology of Low Vision Patients 6
   - Principles of Low Vision Practice 9

2. **Low Vision Examination** 13
   - Visual Behaviour 14

3. **History Taking** 18
   - Goal Setting 21

4. **Visual Acuity Test** 23
   - Factors Affecting Visual Acuity Test 24
   - Measuring Distance Visual Acuity 26
   - Near Vision Acuity Test 32
   - Problems with Projection Chart 35
   - Recording Visual Acuity 35
   - Predicting Near Vision Acuity 36
   - Predicting Reading Add 36

5. **Low Vision Refraction** 39
   - Objective of Low Vision Examination 40
   - Differentiating Factors 41
   - Refraction Procedure 43
   - Application of Different Tools in Low Vision Refraction 49
   - Color Vision Test 51

6. **Patient Counseling** 54
   - Traits of an Effective Counselor 56
   - Components of Effective Low Vision Counseling 62

7. Visual Field Examination 66
- Objective of Visual Field Test 66
- Types of Visual Field Defects 67
- Tests for Visual Field Defects for Low Vision Patients 68

8. Contrast Sensitivity and Glare Test 79
- Contrast Sensitivity 79
- Need for Contrast Sensitive Test in Low Vision 81
- Methods for Contrast Sensitivity Assessment 81
- Tests Charts for Contrast Sensitivity Test 82
- Glare Test 84

9. Common Causes of Low Vision 87
- Achromatopsia 87
- Age-Related Macular Degeneration 88
- Diabetic Retinopathy 90
- Toxoplasmosis 91
- Albinism 91
- Retinitis Pigmentosa 92
- Histoplasmosis 94
- Stargardt Diseases 95
- Aniridia 96
- Glaucoma 96
- Nystagmus 97
- Optic Atrophy 98
- Coloboma 99
- Cataract 100
- Retinal Detachment 101
- Keratoconus 102
- Hemianopia 103

10. Magnifications 107
- Relative Size Magnification 107
- Relative-distance Magnification 108

Contents

- Angular Magnification *110*
- Projection Magnification *111*
- Power of Magnification *111*
- Predicting Magnification Required *112*

11. Illumination 115
- Sources of Illumination *117*
- Ways to Help Patient with Illumination Control *118*

12. Low Vision Aids 121
- Optical Aids *122*
- Nonoptical Aids *133*
- Spectacle Lenses as Low Vision Aids *139*
- Visual Field Expanding Aids *141*
- Contact Lens as Low Vision Aids *144*
- Advanced Low Vision Aids *146*
- Computer-Assisted Devices *150*
- Assessment for Computer-Assistive Devices *155*

13. Prescribing Low Vision Aids 160
- Prescribing Near Viewing Aids *161*
- Prescribing Distance Viewing Aids *165*
- Prescribing for Visual Field Defects *169*

14. Patient's Training 174
- Training for Distance Viewing Aids *174*
- Training for Near Viewing Aids *177*

15. Orientation and Mobility Training 183
- Functional Orientation and Mobility Evaluation *184*
- Mobility Aids and Technique *185*

16. Low Vision Practice Management 187
- Setting Up the Low Vision Clinic *190*
- Setting Up the Fees Structure *190*

- Referrals *191*
- Letter Writing *192*
- Practice Model *193*
- Patient Recall *194*

Bibliography 195
Index 197

CHAPTER 1

Low Vision

Chapter Outline
- Clinical Characteristics of Low Vision
- Psychology of Low Vision Patients
- Principles of Low Vision Practice

When the defective vision cannot be improved by any medical or surgical treatment, low vision devices may alleviate the patient's visual disability to some extent. Low vision or visually impaired is a term used to describe varying degrees of vision loss that cannot be corrected by medications, surgeries, or conventional glasses.

Vision loss may be due to:
- Decreased visual acuity
- Visual field defect
- Decreased contrast sensitivity
- Loss of color perception

Some practitioners define low vision as a visual acuity of up to 6/24 or worse in the better eye using the best corrected spectacle correction or visual field of 20° or less **(Fig. 1.1)**. However, a more functional definition is that low vision comprises bilateral vision loss that adversely affects the performance of daily activities. The patient has either poor Snellen acuity or poor field of vision or both. With such subnormal vision, the subjects are unable to perform their task.

A low vision patient is one who has impairment of visual functioning even after treatment and/or standard refractive correction, and has a visual acuity of <6/18 (20/60) to light perception or a visual

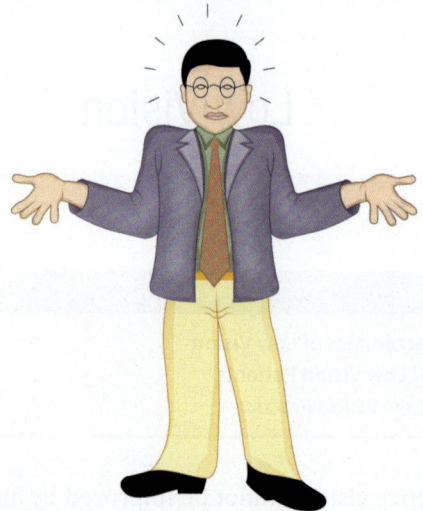

Fig. 1.1: Low vision.

field of <10° from the point of fixation, but who uses or is potentially able to use vision for the planning and/or execution of a task.*

The management of low vision patient is really challenging as it requires patient's cooperation, adaptability, and motivation so that he is ready to use the device. It also requires practitioner's enthusiasm and readiness to spend time with patient to bring him out of the psychological barrier. There are prevailing notions regarding reading at a very short distance or assuming unusual postures for reading. Such notions need to be handled tactfully. Moreover, patient with <3/60 vision can hardly get any benefit. The precise pathology and the lesion are also important to understand as it may affect the type of visual aid which is appropriate.

Low vision care can be considered as a philosophy and vision rehabilitation as the service. The philosophy combined with service work together to make the visually impaired aware of their remaining visual capabilities so that they do not dwell on their impairment. It offers

---

* World Health Organization. Management of Low Vision in Children. WHO/PBL/93.27. Geneva: World Health Organization, 1993.

the patient a real opportunity to regain his visual independence. In practice it has been observed that >95% of people with low vision have some level of useful vision and >90% among them requires reading aids.

CLINICAL CHARACTERISTICS OF LOW VISION

There are many eye diseases that can cause low vision, and can cause various kinds of visual disturbances. The visual disturbances can be grouped as described below.

Loss of Central Vision

Loss of central vision affects the ability to see the objects or people in the direct line of vision. Individual may incur partial loss of central vision or loss ranging from a small sector to the total central loss depending upon the disease and its progression. In such cases, color vision may be affected while peripheral vision remains normal. The individual may also find it difficult to see details and suffer from distorted vision. Usually diseases such as macular degeneration, albinism, Stargardt diseases, toxoplasmosis, and histoplasmosis cause loss of central vision **(Fig. 1.2)**.

Loss of Peripheral Vision

People with peripheral vision loss have various difficulties with independent travel, depending on the degree of vision loss. A person who is just beginning to lose peripheral vision may find himself colliding with the obstacles on the sides, furniture, etc. Some patients with advanced peripheral loss may not be able to detect steps, or other obstacles at all. One form of peripheral vision loss is called "tunnel vision," in which the person sees the world as if looking through a tube with one eye. Retinitis pigmentosa, hemianopia, glaucoma, juvenile diabetes, etc., are the few diseases which can lead to loss of peripheral vision **(Fig. 1.3)**.

Overall Blurred Vision

Overall blurred vision affects the individual's ability to perceive the sharpness of details due to an alteration in the refractive media of

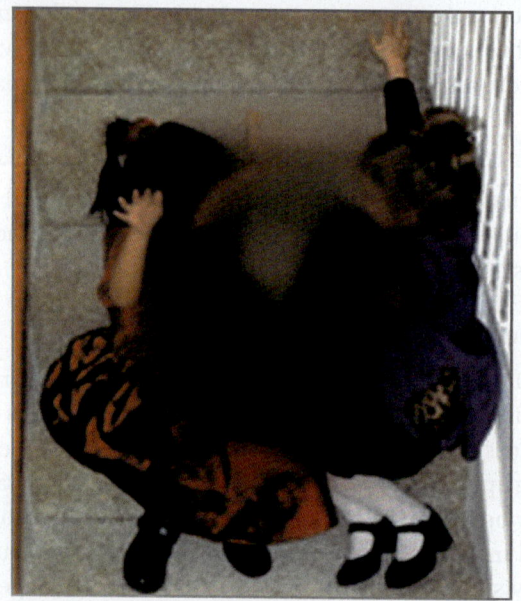

Fig. 1.2: Loss of central vision.

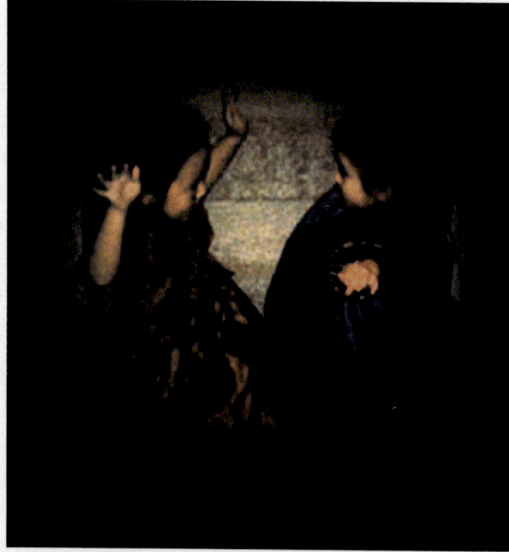

Fig. 1.3: Loss of peripheral vision.

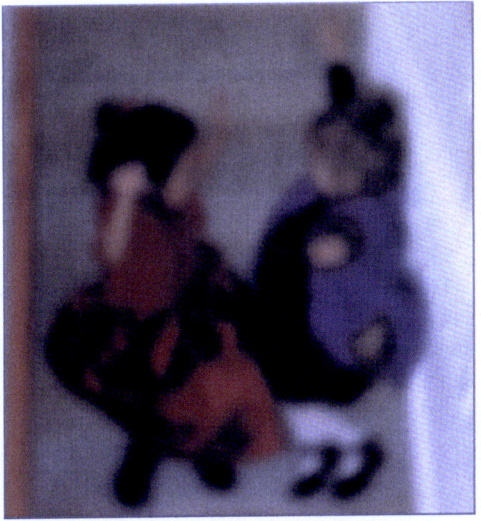

Fig. 1.4: Overall blurred vision.

the eyes. The individual may have blurred vision over the entire field, or over a partial field. The individual may even suffer from double vision, poor night vision, poor contrast, and glare trouble. Congenital, traumatic, and aging cataracts are some of the major reasons for overall blurred vision. Corneal opacities, high myopia, and amblyopia can also lead to overall blurred vision **(Fig. 1.4)**.

Night Blindness

Night blindness refers to the inability to see at night under starlight or moonlight or in dimly lighted areas such as movie theaters. Retinitis pigmentosa, diabetic retinopathy, glaucoma, etc. are a few diseases, which may lead to night blindness.

Light and Glare

Patients with some specific diseases also live in a world where light and glare constantly interfere. Glare reduces the brightness difference and also impairs contrast sensitivity **(Fig. 1.5)**. For patients with retinitis pigmentosa, cataract, etc., walking outside into the sun may result in being overwhelmed by brightness to the point of temporary

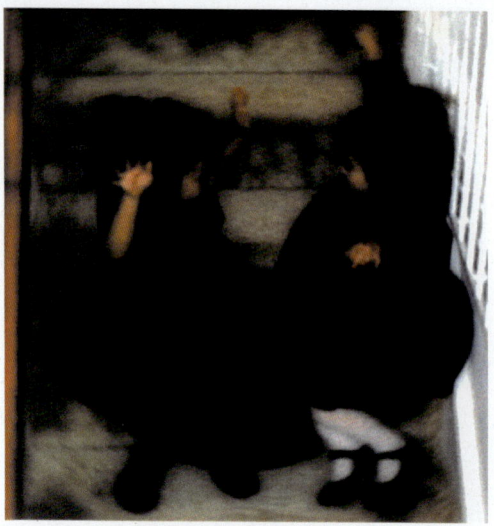

Fig. 1.5: Poor contrast.

Flowchart 1.1: Five stages of grief.

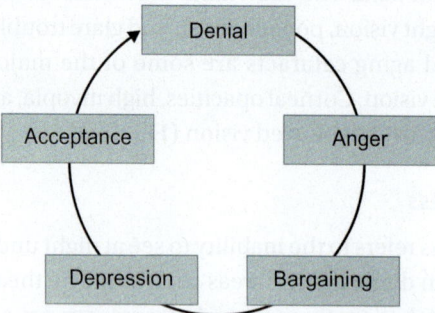

disability. However, light and glare symptoms will vary depending on the degree of damage.

PSYCHOLOGY OF LOW VISION PATIENTS

Most low vision patients usually pass through the five stages of grief that were proposed by Elisabeth Kübler-Ross. These stages are shown in the **Flowchart 1.1**.

The five stages of grief may not necessarily occur in any specific order, but often the patient moves between stages before he becomes a successful user of low vision aids. The first harsh reality that a low vision patient faces is that a single pair of glasses is not enough for his vision. The reality that the patient must hold a magnifying glass and hold materials very close to his eyes is often too much to bear. That is the reason that the first stage is characterized by his quick snap decision that "the low vision stuff is not for me." They at this stage quickly reject any new information or suggestion without taking time to think about some of the new options that are being presented to them. It is almost as if these new ideas are "too big" or "too scary" and often let them soak into their psyche. The reason could be that no one has ever told them about these devices, neither the doctor nor their family member. They are suddenly confronted with unusual devices and things that they have never heard of before. They experience a big "let down psychologically" and for some, this let down is so large that they must first push it away and get out of it. It is like handing somebody a big and heavy pumpkin and telling them to swallow that **(Fig. 1.6)**.

Some patients who cross over stage one will secretly go into their room, put on their reading devices for several minutes, try reading, and then spend the rest of their day acting as if it never happened. And when they feel that even with these devices they cannot see as clearly, they experience their first surges of anger and often take it out on those who are closest to them **(Fig. 1.7)**.

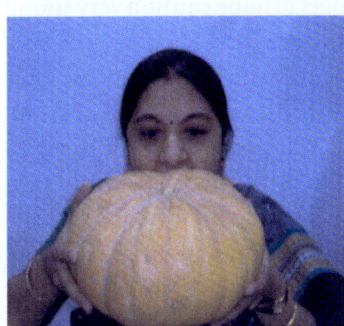
Fig. 1.6: Stage 1.

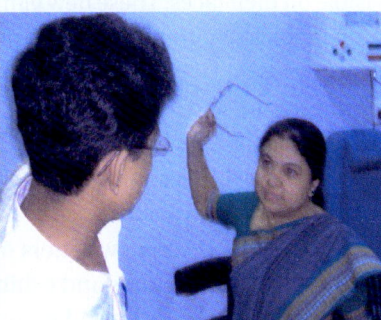
Fig. 1.7: Stage 2.

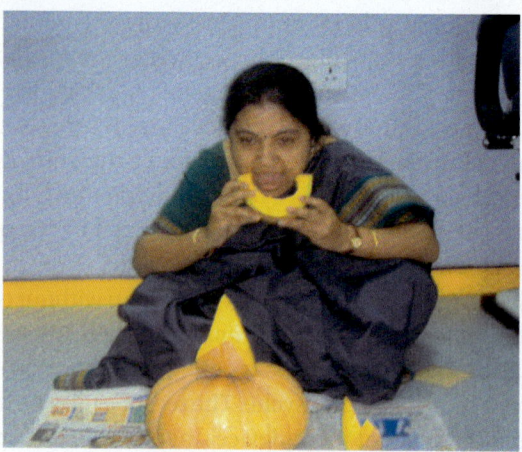

Fig. 1.8: Stage 3.

At the third stage, the low vision patient exposes them to many different low vision options and tools. Now they become a "hard working patient." They start listening to what is being told them and also make an eye contact with the different devices being presented to them. They also ask questions about it. In fact, they start slicing the pumpkin and sample a few bite size pieces **(Fig. 1.8)**. At this stage, some patients often regret to their behaviors that were seen in earlier stage. They start feeling that they need to use the special devices to be independent.

Now glimpses of acceptance and strong glimmers of hope become visible on their faces. These new glimmers of hope can be a very strong motivation to continue trying and refining the process of determining which visual aid works best for the patient in different situations. After feeling strong and confident in the use of one or two visual aids, the patient will look beyond what they currently use and begin to open up to all the possibilities of the various types of devices and want to learn more on how they can be used. They begin to educate themselves by reading low vision newsletters or perhaps attending conventions where low vision lectures and exhibits are presented. Now they start accepting their disability and embrace the use of various low vision devices to become independent functionally. All persons do not reach this stage, but once they meet this stage, they become your ambassador and often reach out to others to help them in any manner.

PRINCIPLES OF LOW VISION PRACTICE

The basic principles of low vision practice are magnification, illumination, and contrast **(Flowchart 1.2)**. Low vision patients do not recognize small and far off targets. When targets are magnified, their image covers more retinal areas, which may have more responsive visual receptors. Thus, a low vision patient is assisted to use his remaining vision. The understanding is that in order for magnification to work for a low vision patient, there must be some areas of the central retina that should function.

Illumination control is essential for low vision patient. A good rule is to give the patient as much light as they can manage without glare. Good room light may yield optimal visual performance for a normal person, but that is not true for eyes with pathology. Most people with low vision have significantly worse function in normal room light condition and encounter difficulty at light levels that a normal individual find acceptable. This is particularly true for patients with photoreceptor dysfunction.

Contrast management is the third important pillar of the low vision practice. Bigger is not always better. Often increasing the contrast of the text is more effective than increasing the size of the text for a low vision patient. People with low vision normally have difficulty seeing

Flowchart 1.2: Three basic principles of low vision practice.

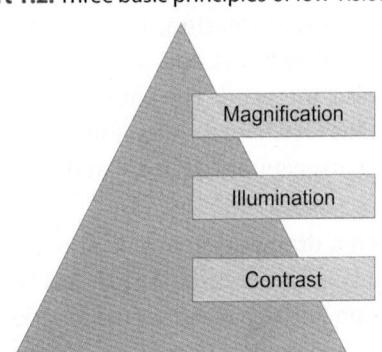

objects or print that has poor contrast. A clear explanation regarding illumination and contrast to the patient can help maximize the function of residual vision.

The service is geared to help patients to maximize the use of residual vision with the help of various optical and nonoptical devices. It does not help the patient to see better in general. It only means helping the patient function better for certain task so that the patient is visually independent. The practitioner makes a list of all the tasks that frustrate the patient in his day-to-day life and work with him to see how they can be managed with the help of various aids. There is no "quick fix" method or "single magic pair of glass" that will do it for all. Instead, depending on the severity of the vision loss, a typical low vision patient may need three or four different aids to help him manage his various visual tasks.

Another way to understand low vision service is that low vision service cannot "help the bad eye." It helps maximize the use of residual vision in the better eye to accomplish the task. Low vision is not medical service, so going for low vision does not mean that the patient will get treatment to fix his vision. In fact, low vision specialist will not be doing things for you. They will accurately describe their role as someone who can work together with you and guide you on your work. It is a beginning of a lifelong process that continues for the rest of patient's life. As people's needs and vision change, low vision rehabilitation will also change to help adapt and make improvements so that they can maintain their "quality of life" as possible.

Unlike other eye examination, the low vision process can take many hours of directions and hard work—not only during examination but also afterward. The patient has to be motivated to take the responsibility for whatever may be asked to get the maximum improvement. You just cannot "sit back" and expect the doctors to do it all.

There has been a dramatic change in the management of low vision patients during last decade. A shift has been noticed from optics and low vision devices toward visual functions. With this new approach, the management of low vision patients is now thought of as a continuing process, beginning with surgical and medical intervention and proceeding through to the prescription of low vision devices and necessary rehabilitative services. In a tertiary care center, it may also include training by an orientation and mobility instructor. The ultimate objective is to enhance the patient's ability to function as close to the normal as possible, using a variety of strategies.

SELECT THE CORRECT ANSWER

1. A low vision patient has....
   a. Poor visual acuity
   b. Poor field of vision
   c. Poor contrast sensitivity
   d. All of the above

2. Which of the following disease causes loss of central vision?
   a. Macular degeneration
   b. Hemianopia
   c. Diabetics
   d. Glaucoma

3. Which of the following disease causes loss of peripheral vision?
   a. Macular degeneration
   b. Histoplasmosis
   c. Stargardt diseases
   d. Hemianopia

4. Night blindness is commonly seen in patients with …
   a. Traumatic cataract
   b. Retinitis pigmentosa
   c. Albinism
   d. Corneal opacities

5. Which of the following is considered to be the basic principle of low vision aids practice?
   a. The practice helps to improve bad eye.
   b. The practice maximizes the vision in better eye so that the patient can accomplish certain task.
   c. The practice improves vision on Snellen acuity test chart.
   d. The practice helps patient to see better in general.

Answers

| 1. d | 2. a | 3. d | 4. b | 5. b |

SELF-PRACTICING QUESTIONS

1. Explain the five stages of grief that a low vision patient may experience.
2. Explain the visual disturbances produced by visual impairment.
3. Describe the basic principles of low vision practice.

CHAPTER 2

Low Vision Examination

Chapter Outline
- Visual Behaviour

Low vision patients are different from the normal population. The low vision patients are aware of their eye condition. They also know that they have lost the vision which cannot be regained by any means. But when they come to a low vision practice as because someone has referred them, they are skeptical and at the same time expect lot of miracles. It is, therefore, very critical to talk to the patients at the onset and to establish the realistic goals for the low vision examination.

Unlike normal eye examination, low vision examination is not driven to achieve 6/6 acuity on Snellen test chart. The visual goals of low vision examinations are to explore patient's goals and concerns and to address them to the extent possible. Different patients may have different goals and concerns. The practitioner who neglects patient's concerns and goals cannot provide satisfactory low vision rehabilitation. Successful rehabilitation occurs only when the practitioner understands patient's goals and concerns and formulates his goals accordingly. However, the goals must be realistic and the patient must be asked to prioritize his visual goals if he is too demanding. The emphasis is on functional vision examination. Functional vision is the use of vision for specific tasks. It is not related to the measure of distance visual acuity or near vision acuity. A patient may have very poor vision for detailed work such as weaving, carving, or reading but may be able to see and avoid objects so that he can move around safely. Many low vision patients can learn to make better use of their residual vision and can function efficiently with only small amounts of visual information. Functional vision may be improved with refractive correction, low vision devices, or instruction in the use of vision.

VISUAL BEHAVIOUR

The holistic and careful low vision examination ideally begins much before the patient enters the examination room. Observations of visual behaviors of the patient in an unfamiliar environment can provide lot of clues regarding the visual status of the patient's eye. Observations are very important in low vision examination. The practitioner must make a note of his observations before kicking off the actual examination procedures. Using these observations, it is possible to design relevant questioning pattern for history taking and then design and implement the examination and rehabilitation strategies for the patient. This is based upon the hypothesis that the patient has developed these visual behaviors over the period of time because of the effect of his ocular condition. It is important to understand what the patient can do for himself, when he needs some help, or how is his visual behavior different from normal population. **Table 2.1** shows the important visual behaviors that may be observed in different low vision patients.

These observations are very helpful to know a lot about the patient. Before you embark on the comprehensive scope of low vision examination, it is important to strategize the way forward. This is important broadly because of two reasons:

1. Comprehensive low vision examination is a time-taking procedure where patient and practitioner's relationship is built up gradually during the examination process. A typical low vision examination may be conducted over a period of time that may range from one to several sessions in 1 day or more. The examination may be conducted in clinic and also in patient's environment. It may also be done indoors and outdoors to assess the patient's difficulties in multiple environments.
2. It is important to understand patient's motivational level at the onset. When low vision patients arrive for a low vision assessment,

Table 2.1: Visual behaviors of low vision patients.

Visual behavior	Relevance
Downward head tilt	Indicates photophobia and adaptation to prevent the effect of glare
Head turns or tilts to one side	Indicates peripheral field defects, the turn is in the direction of field loss
Frequent head and eye movement	Indicates presence of significant field constriction
Unusual head posture	May indicate the presence of central scotoma
Postural stiffness and maintenance of close proximity to walls or handrails	Peripheral visual field loss
Squinting of eyes	Photophobia and presence of refractive error
Erratic eye movement	Lack of central fixation or central scotoma
Eye poking	Discomfort in an irritated eye
Soiled clothing or missing buttons	Possibility of difficulties in the area of activities of daily living
Disheveled, fatigued appearance	Serious systemic disorder

they often talk about the experiences of their previous eye examination. Often they put up their apprehensions and resist accepting the fact that there is a possibility of using residual vision for functional visual independence. "My doctor just dilated me and took lots of pictures and he said that nothing can be done to improve the vision further." These are the common comments that are most commonly heard in the low vision practice. If these apprehensions are deeply rooted, they create a big obstacle in the low vision rehabilitation. The practitioner must spend some time with the patient, make complete effort to remove such perception, and take the process step by step.

Once the patient enters the examination room, low vision care can be offered in multiple models. It is important to design your own

Flowchart 2.1: Preliminary tests for initiating the low vision examination.

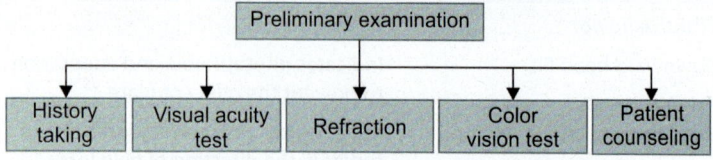

Flowchart 2.2: Specialized procedures for low vision examination.

practice model, including the tests that you would be conducting for your patient, sequences in which you will apply them, your exit protocol and service re-entry. There are diverse ways in which effective services can be provided. The author designed his practice model to suit his private practice and also to make it rewarding professionally. It was designed in the following manner:
- Preliminary examination
- Specialized examination

Preliminary examination procedures were basically to set the goals, direction together with and patient counseling that would allow the author to achieve the desired results. He normally would apply three tests that could allow him to get into visual status of the patient's eyes and followed by patient counseling before getting into the extensive stage of specialized care. The flow of procedures usually includes the following tests as shown in **Flowchart 2.1**.

Specialized examination for evaluating the low vision patients varied depending upon patient's chief concern and his visual conditions. They were all subject to goals and objectives as set at the initiating stage. However, the three procedures as shown in **Flowchart 2.2** were most commonly applied for almost all patients.

SELECT THE CORRECT ANSWER

1. What is the primary goal and objective of low vision examination?
    a. To achieve the 6/6 visual acuity on Snellen test chart.
    b. To bring the focus of the object on to the retina.

c. To address the patient's concerns and expectations to the extent possible.
d. To achieve the practitioner's own objective of clinical practice.

2. During the patient's visit to the practice, a low vision practitioner observes that the patient invariably keeps his head tilted downward. What does it indicate?
   a. It indicates loss of peripheral vision.
   b. It indicates photophobia.
   c. It indicates presence of refractive error.
   d. It indicates that the patient has discomfort because of irritated eyes.

3. During the patient's visit to the practice, a low vision practitioner observes that the patient invariably maintains close proximity to side walls while approaching the examination room. What does it indicate?
   a. It indicates peripheral visual field loss.
   b. It indicates photophobia.
   c. It indicates reduced visual acuity.
   d. It does not indicate anything.

Answers

| 1. c | 2. b | 3. a |

SELF-PRACTICING QUESTIONS

1. What do you understand by functional vision? How can the functional vision assessment help a low vision patient?
2. Define visual behavior. How can a low vision practitioner derive benefits during a low vision clinical assessment by precise observation of visual behavior of patients in the clinic?

CHAPTER 3

History Taking

Chapter Outline
- Goal Setting

The low vision examination begins with an extensive history. In low vision practice, taking a history is not just going down a checklist of symptoms, instead it should be elevated to a greater level of importance to set up a platform from where the practitioner can know the patient's lifestyle, his chief concerns, his motivations, his areas of interest, his family support, and any other information that may help in the assessment and management. Special emphasis is placed on the functional problems of the patients including a chief complaint and any current problem. Care has to be taken to understand how the patient is functioning and his expectations from the low vision assessment.

History taking is an opportunity to talk to the patient, gain his trust, and know the barriers that may be prevailing in the mind of the patients so that during counseling stage they can be effectively used to motivate the patient to embrace the low vision devices. It is also an opportunity to explain the objectives of the low vision practice and take the mystery and fear out of the examination, so that the practitioner can buy their cooperation.

Every aspect of their lifestyle is under scrutiny—whether it is linked to his eye condition, visual disturbances, mental agony, or family support. The practitioner cannot afford to take anything casually. He needs to be quick to show his empathy toward the patients as it would allow him to gain his participation when he will get into the examination and counseling mode. Once the low vision patient sees a good Samaritan in the practitioner, it would encourage him to talk much in detail about his all previous eye examinations and experiences of using any visual aids, if any, which can be very useful as the assessment procedure progresses.

The low vision patient needs to understand that a visual assessment cannot improve his visual acuity but potential for improvement is enormous in terms of functional vision independence.

In author's opinion, it should not be done in the traditional way or in any preset order. Also it should not be done by the assistant; instead it must be done by the practitioner himself. The practitioner may ask question in any order and may make brief records of the information elicited. He may also discuss his successful case history to demonstrate professional expertise and authority.

Table 3.1 shows the relevant questions that may be asked for the purpose of low vision assessment.

Though the **Table 3.1** gives the exhaustive list of questions that the examiner can ask, he must give special emphasis on the following three questions:

Table 3.1: List of questions for low vision history taking.

Lifestyle aspects	Relevant questions
Ocular and systemic history	• Whether there is a family history of visual impairment? • How frequently the patient is monitored by the eye doctor for his condition? • Any recent changes in vision? • Past history of using any low vision aids • Patient's understanding of his ocular and visual condition • Exploration of systemic health status including activities related to distinguishing pills, self-injections of insulin, monitor of blood pressure, monitor of blood sugar level, etc.
Vocational and educational history	• Can he watch the chalkboard? • Is the student attending a blind school or in a mainstream program? • Does he use large print book? • Are there any computer requirements? • Are there any educational needs? • Is the patient employed or doing any volunteer work? • What are visual requirements for their job?

Contd...

Contd...

Lifestyle aspects	Relevant questions
Distance and near vision	• Can the patient recognize the faces of the family members? • Can he see across the road? • What can the patient read? • What happens when he attempts to read? • Has the patient used talking book? • Is he an avid reader? • What low vision devices have been tried?
Activities of daily living	• Can the patient see television? If so, how close does he sit to watch the television? • How large is the television screen? • How well does he see the color on the screen? • Can the patient move independently? • Does the patient use any kind of cane to move? • What are their visual requirements? • Does the patient run into objects or trip on curbs?
Light and glare	• How does he function in bright sunlight, indoor lighting, and at night? • Whether sunglass is worn? If so, what color and type? • Does he use hat or visor? • Does the light and glare affect the patient's mobility? • Does he face difficulty in changing from different light levels?
Emotional and recreational	• How motivated is the patient? • What kind of family support is available to the patient? • Does the patient have any friends to provide support and help? • How is the patient adapting emotionally? Have there been any signs of clinical depression? • What is done for recreation? • Does the patient have any particular hobby?
Visual concerns	• What are his most favorable activities? • Whether he is able to do it or missing it? • Any specific need

1. What would you like to see well?
2. Out of everything that you want to see what do you miss most?
3. What do you know about low vision?

Direct and clear questioning is the key to derive the relevant information that may help the practitioner to set up the goals and develop an initial sense of prognosis for the successful management and rehabilitation. Based upon history taking, the practitioner may also design individualized assessment strategy for the patient as well as also begin to plan for other necessary intervention. The practitioner should be able to understand patient's response to his visual condition and he should also be able to discern how much time to spend with the patient.

GOAL SETTING

With the case history completely taken, the low vision practitioner develops a fair amount of information about the patient's ocular condition, visual condition, emotional and psychological state of mind, his general health, family support available, and his visual needs. Based upon this information and his own knowledge of disease prognosis, he must sit with the patient and set up the goals for the low vision evaluation before initiating the examination process. Goals have to be realistic and specific. It will ensure a planned way forward that will set up the platform on which the success of complete evaluation can be predicted. Goal setting for low vision evaluation, is a methodical process and should ideally be done following a step-by-step process as explained in **Flowchart 3.1**.

Flowchart 3.1: Step-by-step procedure for goal setting for a low vision patient.

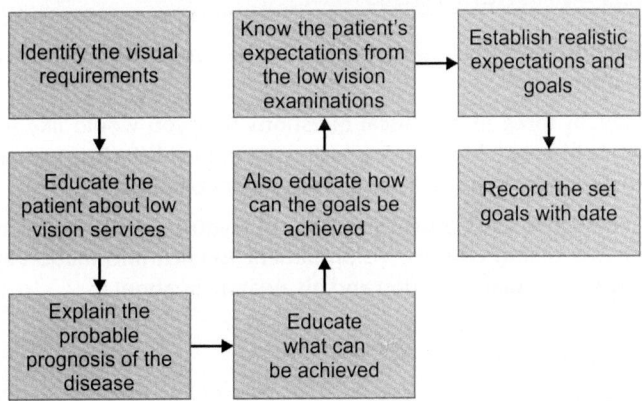

Chapter 3: History Taking

The process of setting goals helps the patient understand the possibilities and builds his interest. He starts participating actively in the hope of seeing the glimpse of first positive outcome of the entire low vision evaluation process.

SELECT THE CORRECT ANSWER

1. Which of the following shows the main purpose of low vision history taking?
   a. Collect patient's information and record them.
   b. Understand patient's environment and lifestyle.
   c. Break the barrier between the patient and the practitioner, understand patient's psychology, and know his areas of concern so that realistic goals can be set for the proceedings.
   d. List the signs and symptoms that needs to be addressed.

2. Which of the following is relevant for goal setting before beginning the low vision examination of a patient?
   a. Know the patient's expectations
   b. Educate the patient about low vision services
   c. Identify visual requirement
   d. All of the above

Answers	
1. c	2. d

SELF-PRACTICING QUESTIONS

1. Why is history taking considered to be very critical in low vision examination?
2. Explain three most critical questions that you would like to ask while history taking of a low vision patient to elicit clues pertaining to patient's keenness to regain visual independence.
3. Explain five most critical questions that you would like to ask while history taking of a low vision patient to elicit information about patient's ocular condition and his awareness about it.

CHAPTER 4

Visual Acuity Test

Chapter Outline

- Factors Affecting Visual Acuity Test
- Measuring Distance Visual Acuity
- Near Vision Acuity Test
- Problems with Projection Chart
- Recording Visual Acuity
- Predicting Near Vision Acuity
- Predicting Reading Add

Visual acuity is the most widely used and most useful clinical measurement for determining the health of visual system. It is the time-dependent measurement of retinal health and is specified by the date on which the eye examination took place. Visual acuity measurement is really challenging in patients with significant functional visual loss. The preferential-looking technique, visual evoked potential, and optokinetic nystagmus testing have been attempted for the objective assessment of visual function. But in practice their application is not very commonly seen. It is measured with the help of various test charts in a clinical environment.

In low vision practice, visual acuity test is normally taken up just after patient's history. Distance and near visual acuity measurements are separately taken. Unaided visual acuity and acuity with existing correction should be taken in the first visit. Both monocular and binocular types of visual acuity are recorded. While testing the visual acuity, it is important to record any eccentric visual angle that the patient resorts to. The examiner should never assume that the patient will have same eccentric visual angle for both distance vision and near vision.

Table 4.1: Adaptive strategies for visual impairment.

Functional deficit	Intervention
Low vision	Instruct the patient to use assistive technology aids and lighting changes so that he can navigate successfully
Visual field loss	Instruct the patient in head turning and scanning techniques. Assess for prism glasses

Flowchart 4.1: Factors affecting visual acuity test.

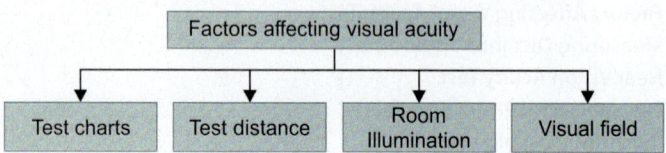

The results of visual acuity tests serve the following purposes:
- To create the baseline information based upon which the entire course of low vision management for a patient is established
- For calculating patient's magnification needs
- Monitor progression of disease and changes in visual abilities as rehabilitation progresses
- Documentation of visual status which can be effectively used for patient counseling.

Since there is no cure of low vision, all interventions aimed will be adaptive in nature (**Table 4.1**).

FACTORS AFFECTING VISUAL ACUITY TEST

Flowchart 4.1 shows the factors that affects the visual acuity measurement for low vision patient.

Test Charts

Traditional test charts are not ideal for low vision patients as there are only a few optotypes available below the acuity level of 20/80. These optotypes are usually the variations of E, which can be easily memorized. The result is often incorrect record of acuity.

Psychologically, if a patient reads only one largest letter on a chart, there may be a feeling of hopelessness. Moreover, it does not allow the examiner to gain an accurate understanding of visual limitations and abilities. There is a large change in size of optotypes, especially at lower acuity level. There are not much steps between 20/100 line and 20/200 line. The change leaves significant gaps in visual acuity level that cannot be quantified. Projection charts have their own limitations. The luminance level of this chart is generally fixed which cannot be changed during patient evaluation. The contrast is poor, especially in older models. The contrast level also varies with the age of the bulb and quality of the screen. It is difficult to measure acuity at various distances with projector chart as the projected image is blocked when the patient walks up to the screen.

Test Distance

Visual acuity with the chart may be recorded at any distance for low vision patient. The test charts can be placed at 4, 3, 2, and 1 m. The practitioner may begin the initial testing at 3 m and ask the patient to read the largest optotype. If the patient finds it difficult to identify, he may reduce the distance and bring the chart closer to the patient gradually. If the patient responds with correct answer, he may proceed through the smaller letters until he misses several letters on a line. The last recognized line would indicate the patient's acuity. Each chart lists a number for the line which is then written as denominator and the testing distance as the numerator which can be further converted to Snellen conventional fraction.

Room Illumination

Room illumination control is essential for low vision patient. The room illumination system should be rheostat mechanism so that variable levels of illumination are possible to duplicate the patient's preferred levels of illumination. The field of illumination should be uniform and glare free. The effect of glare onto an acuity chart can result in a significant underestimation of visual acuity. Internal illuminated charts are useful in the elimination of glare.

Table 4.2: Effect on visual acuity test in visual field loss.

Traits of visual field loss	Effect on visual acuity test
Central scotomas	Visual acuity response will vary depending upon viewing angle, will show higher acuity when letters are isolated
A patient with embedded eccentric fixation angle	Will show more consistent responses
A patient with recent onset of ARMD	Will show inconsistent responses
Hemianopic visual field defects	Will omit beginning or end of a line of letters

(ARMD: Age-related macular degeneration).

Visual Field

Most low vision patients also have varying degree of visual field loss which can produce significant impact during visual acuity test. **Table 4.2** summarizes the effect of visual field loss on the visual acuity test.

MEASURING DISTANCE VISUAL ACUITY

The measurement of distance vision is taken to assess how the patient reacts to visual clues in the everyday environment. However, there is always a difference between visual performances as seen in real life from those of the clinical recording. In clinic the patient is asked to read specially designed eye charts within a setup of controlled environment. Allow the patient to sit in a comfortable chair and to be as relaxed as possible with the head and eyes positioned as the patient wishes. Begin the initial testing of each eye by moving within 2 or 3 feet of the patient and showing the largest number or letter on the chart. If the patient responds with correct answer, back away slowly until the patient indicates it has faded away or 10 feet distance is reached. Proceed through the smaller letter until the patient has missed several letters on a line. The last recognized target would indicate the patient's acuity. Take a light meter reading of the reflectance on the chart and overall room lighting.

Snellen Chart

The commonly used charts to record distance visual acuity are described below.

Snellen Chart

The Snellen acuity chart (**Fig. 4.1**) can be used at various distances such as 4, 3, 2, and 1 m, for the low vision subjects and the data can be converted to the Snellen conventional fraction. For example, a person who can read the letter size of 6 m when the chart is at 4 m, his acuity would be recorded as 4/6. Now in order to translate this to standard Snellen acuity in feet, multiply the top by a number to get 20 and then multiply the bottom by the same number. In the above example if we multiply the top by 5, we get 20. So acuity of 20/30 is recorded. It is important to add the term "equivalent" after the visual acuity.

$$\text{Snellen's acuity} = \frac{\text{Test distance}}{\text{Letter size read}}$$

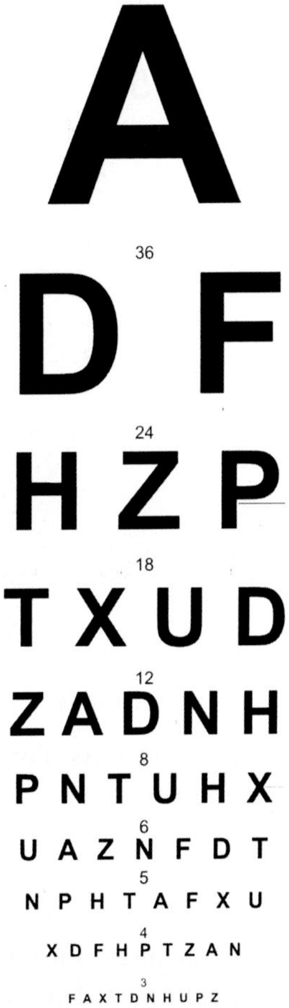

Note that the letter size is a physical characteristic of the letter and does not vary with the testing distance. It is important to note that the units of measurement must be consistent. This means that if a test distance in feet is used, a letter size must be used in feet only. If the test distance is recorded in meters, the letter size must also be recorded in meters.

In practice it has been observed that Snellen chart is not very accurate a very low visual acuity as the patient sees only the letter "E," whereas there are test charts wherein, the patients see many more lines of letters, rather than just the big "E."

Fig. 4.1: Snellen chart.

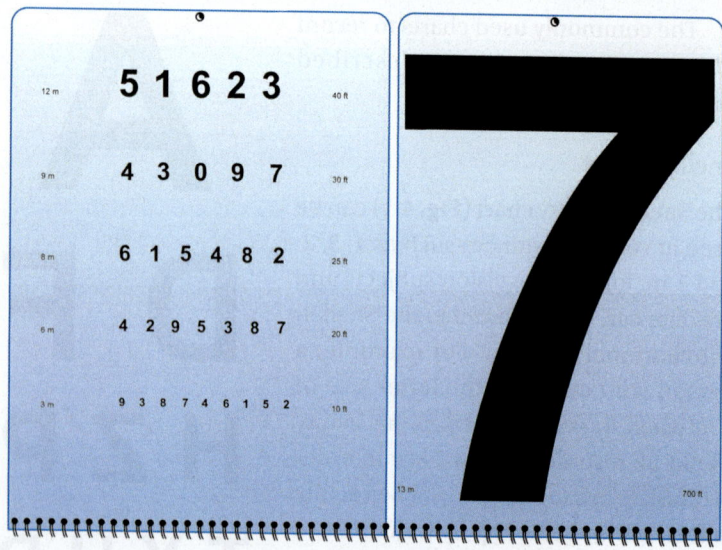

Fig. 4.2: Feinbloom charts.

Feinbloom Charts

Feinbloom charts **(Fig. 4.2)** are very useful to record visual acuity in patients with impaired vision. It is a handheld chart in a spiral bound with flip type book. It contains numbers ranging from 20 to 700 feet size. The advantages of Feinbloom charts are as follows:
- High contrast
- It can measure acuity up to 1/700. Test distance can vary and acuity can be recorded accurately.
- More sensitive at lower level of vision
- It provides a psychological advantage as almost all low vision patients can identify some target number before reaching their visual limit.

Bailey and Lovie Charts

There have been many efforts to improve the design of the Snellen chart. Bailey and Lovie in 1976 proposed a set of principles for the design of visual acuity chart:

- The same numbers of letters at each size level, i.e., five letters in each row, were proposed. Thus, the sizes of the letters become the only significant variable when changing from one size level to the next.
- A logarithmic size progression in a constant ratio from one size row to the next.
- Spacing between the letters and between the rows proportional to the letter size.
- Equal or similar average legibility for the optotypes at each size level.
- Bailey and Lovie logMar chart is a direct chart and cannot be used with the mirror.

Along with these chart design principles, they also introduced the clinical scoring of visual acuity in logMar units as well as a method for giving equal additional credit for each additional letter correctly read.

Optotypes

Sloan and the British letter families are widely used today for visual acuity charts. Both consist of 10 letters that were originally selected within each family. They show small variations in their legibility. The Sloan letters are C, D, H, K, N, O, R, S, V, Z and dimensions are 5 × 5. The British letters are D, E, F, H, N, P, R, U, V, Z and their dimensions are 5 × 4. Bailey and Lovie designed their logMar chart with the British letters. ETDRS chart used Sloan letters. Visual acuity scored with the British letter charts is more reliable than with Sloan letters.

Chart Design

Although spacing between letters and rows within a chart influences the visual acuity score, the choice of spacing ratio is arbitrary. Clinically, it has been observed that letters legibility is increased if they are widely separated. Bailey and Lovie designed the space between adjacent rows and between letters equal to the letter width.

Test Distance

The logMar charts are designed for 4 m direct distance and its letter subtends an angle of 5 minutes of arc at 40 m. Reading the top row at 4 m earns a score of 4/40 which is equivalent to 20/200 or 6/60 in Snellen fraction and logMar value of 1.0. It can be used at 2 m and 1 m also. When used at 2 m, the acuity for the top row has to be recorded as 2/40 and if used at 1 m, it has to be recorded as 1/40, which can be considered equivalent to 10/200 and 5/200, respectively.

Recording Visual Acuity Score

When the acuity is tested on the logMar chart, it is assumed that the patient always has got some score. For example, if he cannot read the letter of 6/60 row, it has been assumed that he could read 6/76 where the LogMar value is 1.1. If the visual acuity has been recorded in logarithmic unit (logMar or VAR), each letter can be assigned a value that is added to the score, when the letter is read correctly. On the chart with five letters by row and the size progression of 0.10 log units, each letter can be assigned a value of 0.02 logMar units. So for each additional letter read, 0.02 is deducted from the logMar score. For example, a patient reads 6/60 row at 4 m, the LogMar value is 1.0. He tumbles in the next row where he can read only three letters, the acuity in this case can be recorded as 1.00–0.06 (0.02 × 3) = 0.94. Thus, letter by letter acuity recording is possible.

Testing Procedure

The first column of the LogMar chart (**Fig. 4.3**) gives the actual letter size in metric notation. 40 M for the top row and is followed by 32 M, 25 M, and so on. The second column gives the conversion to Snellen equivalent. The purpose of this column is to allow us to quickly convert without multiplying, a metric acuity to a Snellen acuity that represents the same visual angle. The number printed in the second column is to be used as denominator of the Snellen fraction with 20 in the numerator if the test is done at 4 m, 10 in the numerator if the test is done at 2 m, and 5 in the numerator if the test is done at 1 m. This is where a common error occurs. It is sometimes understood that the second column is the letter size. It is not so. The first column gives the actual letter size in metric notation. For 40 M for the top row, the correct letter size of this row in feet would be 130 feet and not 200 feet. We cannot place

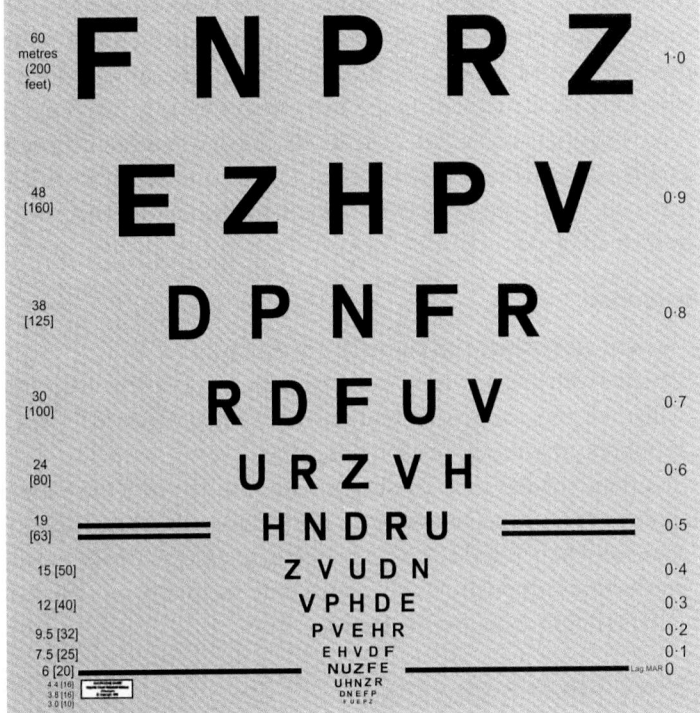

Fig. 4.3: LogMAR chart.

this chart at 10 feet and record acuity of 10/200 for the top row or place it at 5 feet and record 5/200 for the top row. The actual correct acuities would be 10/130 or 5/130. This chart is designed to be used with metric acuities and it should be used in this way. The instruction given on the bottom of the chart gives the procedure for writing the Snellen equivalent of the metric acuity. The conversion table shows:
- When testing is done at 4 m, the numerator of the Snellen fraction is expressed as 20, e.g., –20/200
- When testing is done at 2 m, the numerator of the Snellen fraction is expressed as 10, e.g., –10/200
- When testing is done at 1 m, the numerator of the Snellen fraction is expressed as 5, e.g., –5/200

One interesting point is that 2 m test distance allows the conversion to Snellen equivalent very easily. Just add a zero to the top and bottom number of metric fraction, i.e., 2/32 metric, thus becomes 20/320 in Snellen feet. The 2 m test distance also gives us more acuity range for the low vision patient, i.e., 20/20 to 20/400 Snellen equivalent, instead of 20/10 to 20/200 range when used at 4 m. In addition, it is easier at point to the chart and work with the patients when the chart is 2 m away instead of 4 m.

Advantages

The advantages of logMAR charts are as follows:
- Patients with the low vision can easily follow the pattern of the lines with their consistent presentation of five equally spaced letters, or numbers, or symbols in each line.
- Standard Snellen chart underestimates the acuity of the patients in the critical range between 20/100 (6/30) and 20/200 (6/60).
- Patients when tested at 2 m with logMar chart experience positive sense of accomplishment because they see many more lines of letters (rather than just the big E).

NEAR VISION ACUITY TEST

With the corrected distance prescription in the trial frame and required addition in it, the near visual acuity is measured at 16 inches (40 cm) monocularly and binocularly using special reading charts with optimal illumination. The smallest line read accurately is recorded. Ability to read the print is a function of the size of the retinal image for a patient with low vision. The retinal image increases in size as material is brought closer to the eyes. A low vision patient usually brings the material closer to the eyes. But the near acuity tested at 40 cm is directly related to the power of the addition. Various special reading charts are available for low vision patient, such as:
- MN read acuity chart
- Lighthouse near test chart

MN Read Acuity Chart

The MN read acuity charts (**Fig. 4.4**) are continuous text reading acuity charts for testing both normal and low vision subjects, which

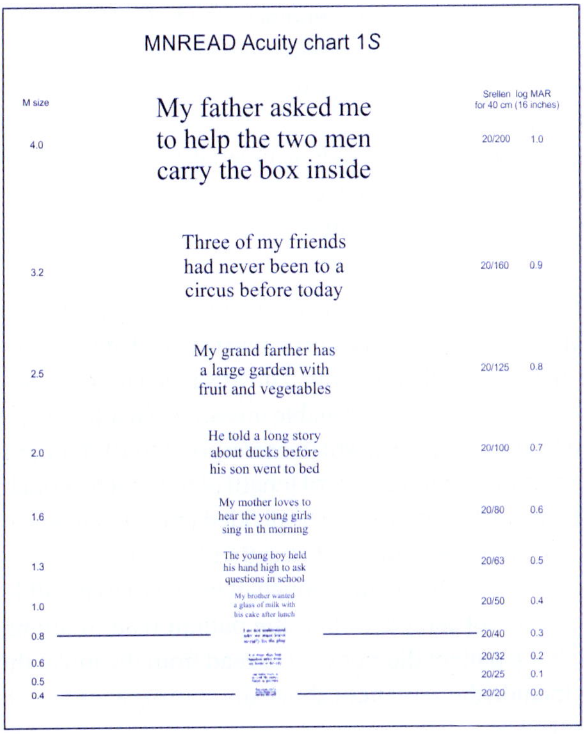

Chapter 4: Visual Acuity Test

M size	MNREAD Acuity chart 1S	Snellen for 40 cm (16 inches)	log MAR
4.0	My father asked me to help the two men carry the box inside	20/200	1.0
3.2	Three of my friends had never been to a circus before today	20/160	0.9
2.5	My grand farther has a large garden with fruit and vegetables	20/125	0.8
2.0	He told a long story about ducks before his son went to bed	20/100	0.7
1.6	My mother loves to hear the young girls sing in th morning	20/80	0.6
1.3	The young boy held his hand high to ask questions in school	20/63	0.5
1.0	My brother wanted a glass of milk with his cake after lunch	20/50	0.4
0.8		20/40	0.3
0.6		20/32	0.2
0.5		20/25	0.1
0.4		20/20	0.0

Fig. 4.4: MN read test chart.

incorporate the modern principles of eye chart design. The chart was developed at Minnesota Laboratory for low vision patients. It contains a progression of 19 sentences in decreasing size print on two sides of a light weight card. It allows measurement of near acuity at the standard viewing distance of 40 cm (16″), with print size ranging from 1.3 to –0.5 logMar, in 0.1 logMar increments. Each sentence is 60 characters long arranged in three lines of text.

Testing Procedure

- The chart should be evenly illuminated so that no shadows or glare will interfere with reading.
- The print size and marking on the chart are designed for a testing distance of 40 cm (16 inches). However, if the chart is used at other distances, the viewing distance must be measured.

- Patient should read the text sentence aloud, starting from the top of chart or from several steps above their previously recorded acuity.
- Mark on the score sheet any words that are missed or read incorrectly.
- Patient should continue reading the smaller sizes until they cannot read any words in a sentence.
- Encourage the patient to guess even where they believe the words are unreadable.

Calculating reading acuity: An estimate of reading acuity is given by the smallest print size at which the patient can read the entire sentence without making significant errors. The MN read chart can be used to provide a more sensitive and reliable measure of reading acuity. Each sentence has 60 characters, which correspond to 10 standard length words, assuming a standard word length of 6 characters (including a space). Thus, each sentence can be divided into 10 smaller parts, and acuity can be measured to the closest 0.01 logMar.

- After the patient has read as much of the chart as possible, count the number of sentences that the patient read or attempted to read. If the patient did not start to read from the top of the chart, then include the sentences above the starting level as if they had been read.
- Count the number of words that the patient reads incorrectly.
- Calculate reading acuity (in logMar) using the following formula:

$$\text{Acuity} = 1.4 - (\text{sentences} \times 0.1) + (\text{errors} \times 0.01)$$

Lighthouse Near Test Card

The second edition of the Lighthouse near acuity test is a reduced version of Ferris-Bailey chart, which is calibrated for 40 cm (16 inches) viewing distance. Nonstretchable 40 cm chord with a ball is attached to the chart to facilitate maintaining test distance. The main feature of this chart is that it provides a guide for selecting dioptric power of reading addition based on test results at two test distances.

Reading is a complex task. It requires a larger functional area to recognize an entire word rather than a single letter. It also involves some more visual skills, for example:

- Fixation to guide appropriate scanning along the line
- Proper image formation and also image detection which brings the topography of the retina into play
- From a functional point of view, testing with continuous text is more informative than testing with a miniature letter chart

However, in real life, reading is undertaken with test of varying quality and contrast, such as newspaper print and the patient may not be able to read as well as suggested by the standardized near vision testing. Therefore, it is necessary to evaluate the use of the recommended low vision aids with the patient's desired reading material.

PROBLEMS WITH PROJECTION CHART

Projection chart in low vision practice is not very useful as they are associated with following problems:
- Less contrast
- No acuity level between 20/100 and 20/200, between 20/200 to 20/300 and 20/400
- Only one letter for acuity of 20/200 to 20/300 and 20/400
- Presented at 20 feet—which is too far a distance for many visually impaired patients to maintain fixation
- Projected charts are not recommended for disability determination.

RECORDING VISUAL ACUITY

In low vision practice, it has no meaning recording visual acuity as FC (finger count). It is not only demoralizing for the patient but also of no use clinically for further management. The practitioner records the acuity in standard fraction or as given by specific charts. Besides, the examiner also makes a note of his observations while recording visual acuity. Some of the important observations that may be recorded are:
- Visual acuity should ideally be recorded in low vision practice together with test distance, illumination level, and test chart used with a note of eccentric viewing, if observed.
- If the visual acuity improves by isolating letters, a note should be mentioned in the record.

- Omission of letters, losing of path while reading test charts should also be recorded. This is helpful information for instructing the patient in the use of optical devices.

PREDICTING NEAR VISION ACUITY

Although near vision task is more complex and reading text is altogether different than identifying letters, it has been tried to predict reading performance from the knowledge of distance visual acuity. The idea has been based upon the principle of Snellen fraction at 6 m distance. The denominator of the recorded distance acuity is divided by 3 to know the N point size of which can be predicted to be read at a distance of 25 cm. For example, if distance acuity recorded is 6/60, then near visual acuity can be predicted to be 60/3 which is 20 which denotes the N-point print size that the presbyopic patient can read at 25 cm with required reading add.

PREDICTING READING ADD

Before evaluating a low vision patient with various optical aids, one should know the strength of the first lens reading add that can be tried with the patient. There has been a lot of effort to provide first reference to required reading add by establishing a relationship between distance visual acuity found with the Snellen chart and the ability to read at a close distance. The objective is to provide the possibility of prescribing appropriate reading device based on distance vision. However, this is more like a theoretical principle. In practice, the patient must be evaluated with the lenses in place using his desired reading material and lenses should be changed until the patient goal is achieved. There are various methods, the most common among them are:
- Kestenbaum rule
- Lighthouse method
- Reciprocal of vision

Kestenbaum Rule

The best corrected distance acuity is used as the basis to predict the reading add. For example, imagine a patient best corrected visual acuity for distance is recorded as 20/200. To predict the reading add, use the reciprocal of 20/200 which is 200/20 which is +10.00 D. The number denotes the dioptric value of add power. The point of concern is distance visual acuity is the poor predictor of near visual acuity.

Lighthouse Method

The Lighthouse near acuity test charts are used that gives the predicted reading add directly from the chart itself. For example, a patient age of 54 years is given the test chart to hold at a distance of 40 cm and +2.50 add is placed over his distance correction. The patient reads as far down the chart as possible. The predicted add for 1 M or 20/50 at 40 cm is then read on the right hand side of the chart beside the last line read. The test is done monocularly and generally the weaker of the two predicted adds is the starting add.

Reciprocal of Vision

The required reading add is calculated based upon patient's best corrected distance acuity and actual desired near acuity level. For example, imagine a low vision patient's best corrected distance acuity is 20/200 and the patient intends to read text the Snellen equivalent of which is 20/40 at 16 inches. The reading add can be predicted as follows:

Predicted Reading Add = (Distance Measured Snellen Denominator/Near Desired Snellen Denominator) × 2.50

In the above example,

Predicted add = (200/40) × 2.50
 = 5 × 2.50
 = +12.50 D

SELECT THE CORRECT ANSWER

1. Which of the following is not the objective assessment of visual function?
    a. Preferential-looking technique
    b. Visual evoked potential
    c. Optokinetic nystagmus testing
    d. ETDRS chart

2. Which of the following factors does not affect the visual acuity test for a low vision patient in the clinical set up?
   a. Test distance and test charts
   b. Practitioners attention and engagement with the patient
   c. Visual field status
   d. Visual acuity measuring techniques and procedure

3. Which of the following is important while recording visual acuity score of a low vision patient?
   a. Test distance and letter size
   b. Room illumination level
   c. Eccentric viewing position
   d. All of the above

4. Which of the following reasons has been often cited against the use of Snellen test chart for visual acuity test for a low vision patient?
   a. At lower level acuity, the patient sees only the letter "E" which is not sufficient to provide accurate measurement of visual acuity.
   b. The letter size does not change based on any logarithmic progression.
   c. The spacing between letters is not standardized.
   d. As it can be used indirectly also.

5. The best corrected distance acuity is used as the basis to predict the reading add. Which of the following rule for predicting reading add is based on the above principle?
   a. Kestenbaum rule
   b. Lighthouse method
   c. Reciprocal of vision
   d. All of the above

Answers

1. d   2. b   3. d   4. a   5. a

SELF-PRACTICING QUESTIONS

1. Why visual acuity measurement is very important in the overall management and rehabilitation of a low vision patient?

2. "Visual acuity level is not the most accurate prognostic indicator of successful low vision rehabilitation." Explain.

3. How does visual field defect affect visual acuity measurement?

CHAPTER 5

Low Vision Refraction

Chapter Outline

- Objective of Low Vision Examination
- Differentiating Factors
- Refraction Procedure
- Application of Different Tools in Low Vision Refraction
- Color Vision Test

Refraction in low vision patient is although a time-taking procedure, but yields enormous satisfaction for both patient and practitioner. The patient gets what he could not get from many eye care practitioners and the practitioner gets a satisfaction of doing something great for someone which in turn is followed by lots of blessings and referrals for him. Most of the time the low vision patients are deprived of good refraction because of the two reasons as shown in **Figure 5.1**.

Common Perception

The most common perception that prevails in the minds of most practitioners is that reduced acuity is solely the result of ocular pathology and correction of refractive error in the presence of ocular

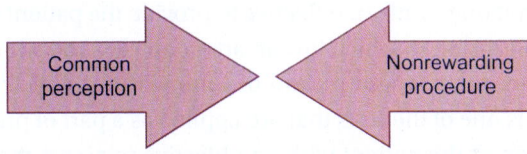

Fig. 5.1: Reasons for inadequate efforts made by eye doctors for low vision patients.

pathology would not result in any change in visual acuity. Driven by this perception, these patients are left to the mercy of medicines and asked to sit back at home with no productive involvement in any work. Another perception that also dominates in their mind is that any acuity around 6/60 is into the category of visual impairment that provides minimal visual information. Therefore, improving visual acuity to a level 6/60 or 6/36 is very often not considered very significant.

Nonrewarding Procedure

A good refraction takes lot of time especially in low vision patients and at the end it may not yield satisfactory results for both patients and practitioners. Besides, patients carry lot of unanswered questions that puzzle the practitioners. This is the reason why they consider it to be nonrewarding both in terms of financial return on time invested as well as patient satisfaction.

OBJECTIVE OF LOW VISION EXAMINATION

A careful refraction is of particular importance in low vision patients because, for reasons mentioned above, they tend to have a high prevalence of uncorrected refractive error. The basic correction of refractive error is important to establish as it forms the basis of the visual acuity test for distance and near and influences the eventual power of the low vision aids. If the refraction is seriously taken up with full commitment, there is always a possibility to have substantial improvement in acuity with conventional lenses, and later options are increased in relation to prescribing optical aids as less magnification will be needed.

Unlike refraction for normal population, refraction for low vision patient is not done with an objective to provide the patient clear and comfortable vision to which he can adapt quickly and which allows him to work for a longer period of time without any symptoms. Instead, it is one of the tests that are applied as a part of preliminary examination of the patient with an objective to assess the residual visual acuity of the patient which can be used more effectively to make the patient functionally independent.

Chapter 5: Low Vision Refraction

The mechanics of refractions applied do not only aim to enhance the visual acuity only but also enables the examiner to establish a baseline acuity on which further enhancement can be achieved by providing low vision aids. The goal of the test is to try and achieve even the little improvement in visual acuity by applying any mechanics whether traditional or unusual to minimize the disadvantage that may arise later in the overall management to achieve patient's visual goals. Therefore, the importance of spending enough time in refraction cannot be ruled out.

DIFFERENTIATING FACTORS

In practice, it has been observed that many times a good refraction is all, that a low vision patient needs. Therefore, it is in the best interest of the practitioner to look at the opportunity to differentiate his practice and approach every case of vision impairment as if the patient needs either +20.00 D or –20.00 D of spherical with 8.00 D of cylinder lens and apply more dynamic methods. It is quite like that the practitioner would need to look at options beyond theoretical methods of general refraction procedure. In general, the factors as shown in **Flowchart 5.1** speak the story of differentiating factors that make the low vision refraction so unique and time taking.

Flexible Test Distance

The standard test distance of 6 m is not very critical. The tests chart may be kept at 3 m distance, instead of 6 m that provides relative distance magnification and enables the patient appreciate more lines on the chart. In case the patient is insensitive to lens changes at 3 m distance, the tests chart may be placed at 2 m or even at 1 m. Eliciting the patient response is the key to quantify the visual acuity. There are other advantages which are as follows:
- When the patient reads more letters or lines, it increases his confidence and he starts responding more enthusiastically.
- Accuracy of test charts at low vision range drops significantly. It is quite likely that the patient is able to see >6/60 but <6/36.

Flowchart 5.1: Low vision refraction, differentiating factors.

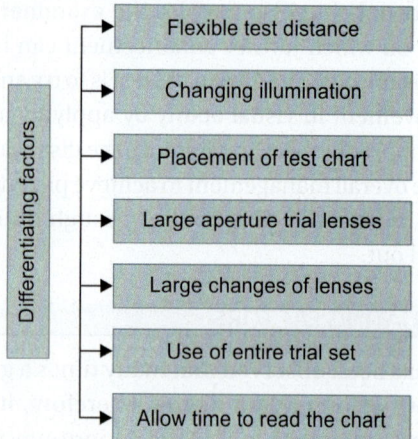

The tests chart at standard test distance cannot quantify the acuity in between distance.

Changing Illumination

Proper illumination is necessary for low vision patients. Light should be adjusted on the printed charts and should not shine on the patient's eyes. Lights coming from oblique sources enter the periphery of eye, thus increase the background illumination and cause glare. Glare decreases contrast and causes strain and fatigue. It is therefore, necessary to control the room illumination. Entire test chart should be uniformly illuminated to minimize the effect of glare. Besides, room light should have rheostat to allow changing room illumination that is comfortable to the patient. Reducing room illumination often improves the comfort and response of achromats or albinos during refraction and provides better visual acuity.

Placement of Test Chart

The placement of test chart is also important for low vision refraction. Ideally the test chart should be placed at the patient's eye level and it should not have propped against the wall. The position reduces glare and also helps altering the test distance.

Large Changes of Lenses

The key to refracting low vision patient is to present the patient with enough of the lens changes to enable him to discriminate the changes in blur. The amount of spherical lens power needed to elicit an appreciable change in clarity or blur is called the "just noticeable difference" or "JND." JND helps the clinician determine the interval between the two lenses that are being compared. The patient would have difficulty responding to smaller dioptric changes than JND at that acuity level. If during the subjective refraction visual acuity improves, JND must be modified to reflect the improvement in acuity. The lower is the acuity, larger will be the JND and vice versa.

Large Aperture Trial Lenses

Use handheld trial frame rather than phoropter as it will allow eccentric head and eye position, most patients would like to acquire.

Allow Time to Read the Chart

The patient's heightened anxiety for subjective test requires that the practitioner should test slowly, giving enough time to discriminate blur. While doing refraction, he must keep trying changing illumination, use filters, and ask him to adopt eccentric viewing so that he could get responses from the patient. There are two extreme types of patients seen in practice—some patients when able to read a line respond with enhanced enthusiasm while there are some patients when they are able to read a line, they pretend very submissively as if the improvement is not very significant.

Use of Entire Trial Set Tools

A patient must be tried with all +/– 20.00 D spherical lenses with all +/– 8.00 D cylinder lenses together with prism, filters, pinholes, and slits to elicit a meaningful result.

REFRACTION PROCEDURE

Like standard clinical refraction procedure, the refraction for low vision patient should also be done in two steps as shown in **Figure 5.2**.

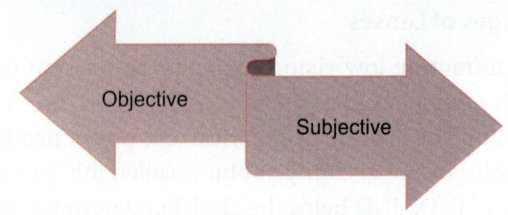

Fig. 5.2: Refraction, a two-step procedure.

Flowchart 5.2: Mechanics of objective refraction.

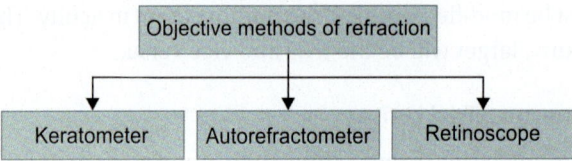

Objective Method

Although objective method of refraction gives a good starting point for the subjective refraction for the regular patients, it is not very effective for a low vision patient as not much information can be elicited by different objective methods for several reasons. However, the importance of objective methods cannot be undermined as it gives a good starting point which can be refined subjectively. There are three common methods of objective refraction as shown in the **Flowchart 5.2**.

Keratometer

Keratometer gives the insights of corneal distortions and indication of the presence of a large amount of astigmatism that may be missed otherwise. This can be used even if the patient has nystagmus. The clinician should attempt to elicit a viewing posture that reduces or eliminates the nystagmoid eye movements and then measures corneal curvatures.

Autorefractometer

Autorefractometer in low vision patients mostly does not work because of several reasons. Small pupils, inadequate fixation, opacities of ocular medias, corneal irregularities, accommodative abnormalities, and ametropia beyond the range are the reasons. Some posterior segment abnormalities reduce the intensity and definition of fundus reflex. Certain geriatric and pediatric patients are difficult to measure because of their inability to keep the head in position and eyes fixated, and patients with Parkinson disease or nystagmus may prove impossible to clinically perform autorefractometry.

Retinoscopy

A skilled optometrist relies on the retinoscope as an invaluable tool to determine the refractive error. But it is usually difficult in case of low vision patient to do retinoscopy because of media opacities, pupillary size and location, and various optical irregularities. However, radical retinoscopy can be performed in situations where reflex cannot be observed due to media opacity with large aperture trial lenses. While performing radical retinoscopy, the practitioner should keep in mind that speed and brightness of the reflex are the functions of the closeness to neutralization. As neutrality is approached, the brightness of the reflex should increase as should the speed of the retinoscopic reflex. Either a spot or a streak retinoscope may be used. The streak facilitates the determination of the major meridian of astigmatism, whereas the spot retinoscope may be more useful in determining the refractive error.

Subjective Method

Because of the ineffectiveness of the objective refraction techniques to provide sufficient information, subjective refraction is more important for patients with low vision. Subjective refraction is the area where the practitioner has to be more dynamic and ready to try all unusual processes. The idea is not to apply the methods of refraction but to elicit some clues on which a meaningful refraction can be performed.

Critical Factor

The subjective refraction should be done with the handheld trial lenses and trial frame and not with phoropter because this allows for eccentric head or eye position most patients require and also the examiner can watch the patient's head and eye movements during the test. If the patient is hidden behind the phoropter, he or she may have to assume an unnatural posture just to see through the instrument, hence unreliable findings may be obtained.

Starting Point

The starting point for subjective refraction is very critical for a low vision refraction. The following options can be looked at:
- Based on the results of objective refraction
- A habitual spectacle prescription
- A Halberg trial clip may be used over spectacle to elicit the changes needed in the previous correction using spherical trial lenses and the results can be used as starting point.
- If no reference as to the refraction is available, then assume each patient has severe myopia or hyperopia with a cylindrical component. Determination of refractive error may be accomplished by bracketing technique, in which plus and minus lenses of equal powers are compared until a favorable response is elicited.
- The same technique may be applied to find cylinder component, by comparing a cylinder lens at the four major meridians to another cylinder lens and so on.
- In extreme case, the practitioner may need to use his best judgment based on patient ocular history and entering acuities.

Procedure

Low vision refraction is not only a matter of asking the patient to discriminate the clarity between two lenses. It is about working with the patient to improve acuity by changing the light levels, testing through filters and using larger changes.

Adjust the trial frame as regard to its temple length, bridge height, pupillary distance, pantoscopic tilt, and vertex distance. Vertex distance is important in the prescription over +10.00 D and –10.00 D. Small error in the estimation of vertex distance creates clinically significant differences in the refractive correction. For example, suppose a myope is refracted at 12 mm vertex distance with –15.00 D and if he is fitted

Chapter 5: Low Vision Refraction

with a glass where the back vertex distance is 8 mm from the cornea, he would be "overminused" by almost a diopter.

The key to refracting low vision patients is to present the eye with enough of the lens changes for the patient to discriminate the changes in blur. The amount of spherical lens power needed to elicit an appreciable change in clarity or blur is called the "just noticeable difference" lens or the JND. JND helps the clinician determine the interval between the two lenses that are being compared and is based on the patient's best visual acuity at 10 feet. To calculate the JND, the denominator of the acuity at 10 feet is divided by 100. For example, if the patient's best acuity is 10/200, the JND will be +&- 2.00D (200/100). The patient would have difficulty responding to smaller dioptric changes than JND at that acuity level. If during the subjective refraction visual acuity improves, JND must be modified to reflect the improvement in acuity. The lower the acuity, larger the JND and vice versa. The JND may also depend on the pathology and individual sensitivity.

The first step in subjective testing is to find the best sphere. Put the starting lens in the back barrel of the trial frame. Direct the patient's attention to a line larger enough to maintain fixation. Present the patient with the JND interval using a plus and minus lens of equal absolute value and ask to compare the clarity.

For example:

Patient X

Entering acuity R.E.: 20/200 L.E.: NLP

Retinoscopy unobtainable

Old glasses unobtainable

JND 2.00 D

Trial frame has no lens in it. Find the best sphere.
- Ask the patient to compare +1.00 Dsph to –1.00 Dsph. Patient states that +1.00 Dsph is clearer. Place +2.00 Dsph in the trial frame.
- Again, ask the patient to compare +1.00 Dsph to –1.00 Dsph, this time with +2.00 D already in the trial frame. If the patient still prefers the plus lens to the minus, replace the + 2.00 D in the trial frame with +4.00 Dsph.

- Again ask the patient to compare +1.00 Dsph to −1.00 Dsph, this time through +4.00 Dsph in the trial frame. If the patient prefers −1.00 Dsph to +1.00 Dsph—this is called reversal and we now know that the best sphere is more than +2.00 Dsph but less than +4.00 Dsph. We can replace the +4.00 Dsph lens in the trial frame by +3.00 Dsph and continue refining the best sphere by letting the patient compare the JND lens in front of the +3.00 Dsph in the trial frame.

Notice that we are determining the best sphere by bracketing around stronger and weaker lenses. In this way refractive error can be arrived quite accurately and reliably in low vision patients. Remember that we are changing the corrective lens in the trial frame, but not changing the +1.00 Dsph or −1.00 Dsph JND lens that the patient is being asked to compare. However, if the acuity improves, the JND may be decreased. For example, in our above case if the acuity improves to 20/100, ask the patient to compare +0.50 Dsph to −0.50 Dsph lens.

Once the best sphere is determined, test the patient for astigmatism. If the K reading or retinoscopy indicates astigmatism, refine axis first, then power using the handheld Jackson Cross Cylinder (JCC), the strength of which is chosen using the same JND rule of thumb. Use ±1.00 D JCC to test the patient in the above example. It is recommended to keep the following set of JCC in the trial set +0.25 D and −0.25 D, +0.50 D and −0.50 D, +0.75 D and −0.75 D, and +1.00 D and −1.00 D. First correct the axis using the handheld JCC and then test the cylinder power by changing with the JND and get a reversal in the same manner. Remember to keep spectacle equivalent constantly while changing cylinder powers. If the patient accepts large changes in the cylinder power, do not hesitate to recheck and refine spherical component to obtain valid findings.

After finalizing cylinder correction, retest for the best sphere with the JND lens. If the keratometry or retinoscopy indicates a spherical (nonastigmatic) error, do not forget to test subjectively for the presence of astigmatism after the best sphere has been determined. Check for the presence of cylinder power with or against the rule, by flipping the JCC in front of the best sphere with its handle oriented at 45° (the power meridians will be at 90 and 180°). If the response indicates astigmatism, place a JND amount of cylinder in the trial frame at the appropriate orientation, adjust the sphere to keep the spherical equivalent constant, and refine axis and power. If the response indicates equal blur on both sides of the flip, the patient has either no astigmatism, or has cylinder axis at 45 or 135° and we must test for the possible existence of this oblique cylinder by changing the orientation of the JCC handle by 45° and flipping again. If the response indicates equal blur on both sides of the flip, we may conclude that there is no cylindrical component. But if the response indicates a preference for oblique cylinder, place a JND amount in the trial frame at the appropriate axis, keeping the spherical equivalent constant, and refine axis and power. After refining cylinder, go back to refine sphere as discussed earlier.

The Snellen numerator of the recorded final best-corrected acuity should reflect the subjective test distance. For example, if the subjective refraction at 1 m is +2.00/–1.50 × 90° and the smallest line read was the 10 M line, record the subjective as +2.00/–1.50 × 90 D, as 1 M/10.

Be sensitive to the patient's heightened anxiety for the subjective test, test slowly and carefully, giving enough time to discriminate blur. Repeated presentations to certain patients are necessary to yield valid results.

Some patients who appear to have "low vision" may actually be in need of a careful refraction only particularly albinos, high myopes, and postoperative lens implant patients. However, it is not always wise to give a new prescription until the patient compares the findings binocularly with the old glasses, not just looking at the vision chart, but also out of the window or down the room.

APPLICATION OF DIFFERENT TOOLS IN LOW VISION REFRACTION

As we discussed earlier that the mechanics of refractions applied in low vision refraction do not only aim to enhance the visual acuity to prescribe a pair of corrective lenses only but also enable the examiner to establish a baseline acuity on which further enhancement can be achieved by providing low vision aids. It is, therefore, quite likely that the examiner may need to look at options beyond theoretical methods of general refraction procedure and use entire trial lens set or others as tools for the purpose of clinical refraction. Some of the important tools that he may apply effectively in low vision refraction are described below.

Filter Lenses

Filters eliminate the strain and discomfort and take away the sparkles, flashing, and other perceptual distortions that some individuals see. Glare can interfere with vision and create discomfort. Filters increase contrast, making it easier to see the letters, words, and numbers while increasing comfort. Wearing the right color for you, in combination with magnification, can increase the length of time you can read and do other visual tasks.

Pinhole

Patients with irregular cornea, whose refractive error cannot be corrected by glasses, can be benefited by using opaque disks with multiple pinholes which provide refractive correction whichever direction the patient gazes. Individuals with macular disease, as well as those with other ocular diseases that affect central vision, may have similar or even reduced acuity when looking through a pinhole. This is because the reduced amount of light entering through the pinhole makes the chart less easy to read.

Stenopaic Slit

The slit is used to help determine the cylinder component of the refractive error. It can also be useful in determining the total refractive error of the patient. However, it should be noted that the patient's choice of the slit position may not always identify the axis of astigmatic correction. In some patients, it may represent an area of unobstructed vision. It should be clearly understood that the slit is helpful only as a guide to the subjective refraction.

Prisms

Prism can be used very effectively during low vision patient's refraction for image relocation which may increase the acuity significantly. The technique is very useful in patients with central scotoma in which case the image is shifted from fovea to parafoveal region. The power and orientation of prism is determined by trial and error method. Refraction is performed after the prism orientation is identified. Prism is placed with its base in the direction of the functional retina. Care must be taken to ensure that the patient looks directly ahead and does not follow the image shift when the prism is used.

Contact Lenses

Contact lenses are often of great value in improving the acuity of the people with distorted corneas, and high refractive errors. Contact lenses are particularly important for people with high refractive error and small fields. Such people must scan to realize a meaningful functional field; if they have to scan behind a thick correction lens, they either suffer the distortion from the lenses or scan with their head to maintain their visual fields in clear part.

COLOR VISION TEST

Many clinicians often ignore to perform color test for low vision patients as most tasks involved in daily living do not depend on a person's color discrimination, and color vision deficiencies, whether hereditary or acquired, cannot be corrected anyway. In spite of this, there are two reasons to consider color test for low vision patients.

Diagnostic Purpose

Color vision tests results in conjunction with other examination findings can sometimes be a valuable part of a diagnostic profile, especially when the etiology of patient's vision loss is uncertain.

Functional

Some patients may depend on color discrimination for certain tasks in their daily life. Knowing which colors are confused may allow the low vision practitioners to counsel the patient on color selection, or on alternate clues or methods of identification, that will help optimize the patient's visual function. Numerous standardized color

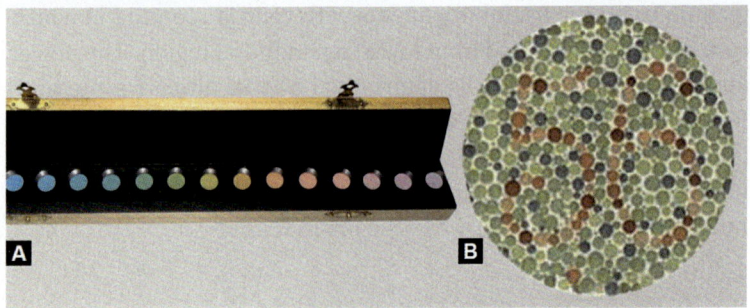

Figs. 5.3A and B: Color vision test types. A. Farnsworth-Munsell D-15; B. Ishihara chart.

tests are available commercially. For patients with low vision, the "Farnsworth-Munsell D-15" test **(Fig. 5.3A)** is a good choice as it is more informative. In this test, 15 colored disks are arranged by hue. This provides a sensitive index of abnormalities of color vision. The pattern of variation from normal also provides information as to the type of color deficiency. If the color vision test is to perform for diagnostic purpose, it must be done monocularly. However, if it is being performed only to see how the low vision patient is functioning in term of confusing colors, it is sufficient to perform it binocularly.

SELECT THE CORRECT ANSWER

1. Which of the following is the true objective of low vision refraction?
   a. A substantial improvement in visual acuity can be realized with conventional lenses that enhances the option to prescribe optical aids.
   b. Bring the image of the object on to the retina
   c. To prescribe a pair of correct optical lens
   d. To provide clear and comfortable vision

2. Which of the following is not the unique feature of low vision refraction?
   a. Flexible test distance
   b. Changing room light
   c. 20 feet test distance
   d. Large changes of lenses

Chapter 5: Low Vision Refraction

3. Which of the following is relevant regarding room illumination in low vision refraction?
   a. Reducing room illumination improves patient's comfort and response in patients with albinism
   b. Light should be directed on to the chart, not shine on the patient's eyes.
   c. Excess light causes glare
   d. All of the above

4. Retinoscopy is not very helpful in low vision refraction because of…
   a. Media opacity
   b. Pupillary size and location
   c. Optical irregularities
   d. All of the above

Answers

| 1. a | 2. c | 3. d | 4. d |

SELF-PRACTICING QUESTIONS

1. How is low vision refraction different from general refraction procedure? Explain.
2. Refraction in low vision patient is very important for successful rehabilitation of the patient. Illustrate.

CHAPTER 6

Patient Counseling

Chapter Outline
- Traits of An Effective Counselor
- Components of Effective Low Vision Counseling

Counseling is a personal and dynamic relationship between two individuals. Counseling aims at helping the patients understand and accept themselves "as they are" so that they can help themselves. Counseling should never be considered same as "history taking." The main objective of counseling is to bring about a voluntary change in the patient. Patient counseling is a very important element of low vision practice and is done to achieve the following three objectives:
1. To give the patient information on the current status of his visual condition, especially with regard to residual vision and how can it be used to become functionally independent.
2. To know the patient understands regarding his own ocular and visual condition and also to understand his readiness to accept the complete low vision rehabilitation program as a way of life, his family support, and off-course financial capabilities. The practitioner understands patient's behavior, motivations, and their feelings.
3. To encourage and develop special abilities and right attitude toward low vision services and also to inspire successful endeavor toward attainment of the objectives of vision rehabilitation program. The goal is to help patients attend their immediate problems and also to equip them to meet future problems.

Most low vision patients are aware of their ocular condition and also to some extent their visual prognosis as they had heard from their ophthalmologists before visiting a low vision practitioner. They know that they have something very serious condition which cannot be treated by any means. But most of them are not aware of the fact that they have something called residual vision with their impairment which can be used effectively to perform certain tasks. Residual vision is the term which is given to usable vision with the impairment, for example, a glaucoma patient who has impaired vision in his peripheral visual field may still have residual vision in the central visual field. Similarly, a patient with macular degeneration whose central vision is lost may still have residual vision in his peripheral visual field. This may sound to them as a new term which provides them with rays of hope and may prompt them to know more about it.

Understanding patient's readiness to accept low vision services as a way of life is really challenging. Two factors influence the decision more than anything else. They are as follows:
- Patient's motivation and his spending power
- Patient's confidence on the practitioner

Vision disabilities of low vision patients have profound effect on their lifestyle and they feel that their independence is slipping away, often leading to depression. The overall effect is observed as poor motivation as they use denial as a defense mechanism for anything that is offered to them as aids. The low vision practitioners have to understand patient motivation's level and encourage them to use what vision they have to enhance the quality of their life. This is definitely time-consuming but this is the key to success. Recognizing the fact that the patients are also clients to whom aids can be sold to make the practice commercially profitable is another truth. When it comes to spending money to buy aids, the low vision patients are selective and skeptical. They always look for cheaper options and do not readily accept costlier aids. Sometimes they also look for experiencing opportunity before taking decision to buy the aids which is very demotivating for the practitioner.

Most patients are willing to spend anything if they develop a feeling of trust and respect for the practitioner. The straight forward implications are that the practitioner needs to inspire the patient. It is not easy because no single thing works. A host of things should be in place. Integrity, commitment, and truthfulness are three building blocks of trust. You need to shape what your patient thinks about you and it has to be insanely patient caring. And it needs to be memorable in the minds of your patient and unique to you. Eventually you will burn you and your practice into your patient's mind. Sometimes trying hard does not work; you need an intelligent approach. On many occasions, the author has successfully used the power of mind game in his practice to drive the patient to use low vision devices. It is a very effective technique that works in difficult situations or with difficult patients or with patients who come with some preconceived notions. It is important that you know how to "hold your own," keep your entire sense organs active and be natural to let the things happen while recommending high value gadgets. Patients themselves will show you the way and you will be able to apply the technique unique to your patient.

TRAITS OF AN EFFECTIVE COUNSELOR

One of the reasons why low vision practice is not rewarding commercially is the fact that most low vision practitioners are neither good counselors, nor they like to spend time in counseling. Caring attitude is critical. Caring involves a deeper level of understanding than the gentle application of science to the amelioration of disease. Although there are lots of factors but in order to be an effective low vision counselor, the practitioner has to take care of following five elements as shown in **Flowchart 6.1.**

Self-confidence

Self-confidence is very critical for being a good counselor as it inspires the patients. The immediate effect of self-confidence can be

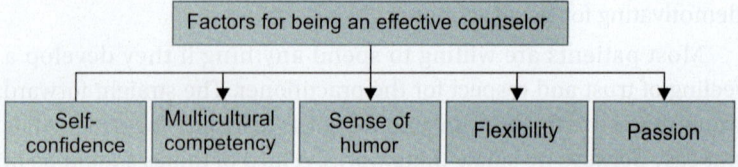

Flowchart 6.1: Factors that affect the ability of the examiner for being an effective counselor.

observed on the body language of the practitioner. Body language is very important way of communication in any face-to-face interaction. Not only it affects how people perceive you, it also has a lot to do with how you feel about yourself. New practitioners are low on self-confidence, whereas experienced practitioners are relatively stronger on self-confidence. The possible reason could be it is being destroyed in the didactic years and is built back in the clinical years as suggested by many researchers. However, lack of self-confidence is often seen in experienced practitioners also. Two possible reasons for their conditions are fear of not knowing and fear of making mistakes. These behaviors have far reaching effect on the practice and affects adversely on our ability to deliver. The practitioner finds it difficult to connect with what he is supposed to do and began to doubt himself. Self-confidence is something that you learn to build up if you keep helping yourself in this challenging environment of the real world. Remember self-care is never a selfish act; in fact, it is more important than helping others. There are simple ways to help yourself—know your weaknesses, appreciate your flaws, and learn from your mistakes, you'll be high on self-confidence.

Multicultural Competency

Low vision patients come from different walks of life and from different background. Cultural competency can help low vision practitioner establish better rapport with their patients, improve level of communication, and develop the ability to approach patient counseling through the context of patient's world. It helps practitioner–patient relationship progress appropriately, ethically and holistically through communication. One of the effective ways is to start counseling identifying your own worldview and personal beliefs and then proceed with acknowledging patient's feelings and ideas. Having open mind to learn new ideas plays an important part in shaping up your professional identity.

Sense of Humor

Humor helps us shaking off things. It helps us see more of our humanity and provides us an opportunity to realize that the world is not always a somber and serious place. It is an effective tool of any interaction and communication. Make sure that your humorous statements should not be offending to the patients or any other person accompanying the patient. Laughter is an essential part of the human experience and it can be effectively taken up even in the therapeutic relationship as a means of expressing thoughts in the unconscious way. Research has found that when working with diverse populations, the practitioner's use of humor can help patients to perceive the practitioner as their ally in the strange or potentially threatening environment of the consulting room.

Flexibility

The practitioner must be flexible while counseling the patient. Flexibility in patient's counseling is defined as the ability to adapt and change the way you respond to meet the patient's needs. You do not stay rigid and stick to a predetermined treatment path when your patients require a different approach.

Passion

A successful low vision practitioner is also very good in the art of persuasion. There are two areas of low vision practice—low vision assessment and prescribing aid to the patient. The low vision practitioner has to face lot of resistance from the patient when it comes to prescribing and dispensing aids. There are several reasons such as patient's apprehension, price, limited application of the aids, and his dependency on family support for fund. The entire scenario is very complicated. The practitioner needs to be passionate for who he is, what he is doing, and what he believes in and it must shout to the world, "I'm here to rule, make my mark in this world and I'll not give up until I achieve my objectives."

In medical practice, one of the very effective ways of learning the art of patient counseling is the experiences of counseling patients. The experiences may be your own or other successful practitioners. The author had recorded several successful patient counseling cases during his practice. One of the interesting cases that he had was of a girl, aged 9 years who was diagnosed albinism with nystagmus. Her

general health was excellent. Her parents came to the author's clinic with a reference of a satisfied patient from his practice only. The girl was last seen by an ophthalmologist who practically denied any help saying nothing much can be done. The author had a comprehensive low vision examination which took two sessions and finally he decided to prescribe her:
- Pinhole contact lenses
- Refractive correction
- Telescopes for reading blackboard in the school
- Environmental control especially illumination and glare
- Use of visor

When the author started explaining them about her prescription, he got immediate resistance from girl's mother as she said, "She had only heard about spectacles, not gadgets like telescopes." The author called them for another session to counsel her mother. The summary of the discussion that happened between the author and her mother was as follows:

Author (with a pleasant smile on face): Your daughter seems very intelligent and smart. Unfortunately, she is suffering from albinism. Albinism is a genetic condition which is characterized by absence of pigments in the body and eyes both. Pigmentation in eye is essential for normal vision. Together with this nystagmus is also present. Distance vision is severely affected but near vision is quite good and there is no visual field defect. As I told you in the beginning when I was talking to you about your general health and eye condition of your daughter at the beginning I categorically told you that low vision services cannot bring in restoration of normal vision but it can certainly help your daughter use her residual vision to her advantage, to study and do her most task independently.

Mother (with little excitement): What is "Residual Vision"? No doctor has told me before about this.

Author (noticing her excitement): Residual vision means central vision is poor due to underdeveloped macula but side vision is excellent which means she can work wonderfully with the telescope that I would like to give her.

Mother (little anxious): Don't you feel that she is too young to use telescope kind of gadget. Moreover, you have also suggested so many others. How will she be able to manage?

Author: Well! That's my concern as well. Had I been in your place, I would have kept aside some of my time for my daughter so that I could take care of her. It is a question of her life. At this stage if she cannot read just because she is not normal visually, her entire life at the later stage will be in dark. I know it is difficult to maintain the regularity. But trust me it is a matter of a few days only. Once she learns the use of telescope and tastes its advantages, she will become responsible by herself. This is what I have seen with my several patients. Difficulties or hesitancies have very short lifespan. You need to understand that she is your daughter and if you don't take care of your daughter, who else will take care of her. As far as number of aids is concerned, you may prioritize. Decide what is important for her and focus on those areas. For telescope you don't need to do much. I'll teach her how to use it. Teaching the use of gadget is a part of the entire package. You only need to ensure that she carries it to her school every day. Just like lunch box that you give her every day, you need to give her telescope also and trust me this is also a short-lived problem. Once she realizes that she can see the blackboard clearly using telescope, she will never forget it thereafter. This is what I have seen in my practice. Many of my patients are using it successfully. Other aids are not very difficult to use.

Mother (seemed little relaxed): What are the cost involvements? Do we have to buy everything together?

Author: The only aid that is a little expensive is the telescope which is very important for her education and career, so unavoidable. Pinhole contact lenses are not very expensive but they are going to reduce your engagement with her as while at home pinhole contact lens together with spectacle will work wonderfully for her to work independently.

Father (candidly): Sir, you were talking about illumination and environment control, what are they?

Author: Patients with ocular albinism usually function almost like a normal person when illumination level is dim and there is no glare in the visual field. Excessive lights are not good for your daughter. There are different ways of reducing the illumination and minimizing the glare effect. You may maintain dim light in general at your home and also save on electricity cost. Or, you may get a pair of tinted lenses which she can use indoor and outdoor both. Next time when you plan painting your flat, use matt finish paints.

Father (wrapping up): So finally, what do you suggest?

Author: You have to decide. How would you like to go about? You must understand that this is the beginning of our relationship. With time things will change. Your daughter's needs will change. New tools will be introduced. Ocular condition may also change. You may need to change the aids and in that situation whatever, you'll take today, may not be of any use then.

Father: Allow me some time. I'll discuss with my wife and join you back in ten minutes.
(Nearly 10 minutes later, they came back)
After a pause,

Mother: Sir, how much it would cost us?

Author: The total expenditure of entire rehabilitation program would include consultation fee, cost of telescope and contact lenses and training fee.

Mother: What is this training about?

Author: Good question. Your daughter has to be trained on several elements of program including use of telescope, viewing technique, care and maintenance of contact lenses. She would not be able to use them otherwise. All of these services would take lot of chair time.

Mother (with little apprehension): Sir, we're from middle class family. We cannot afford a very high cost.

Author: Don't worry. We have different payment modes. I'll ask my receptionist to explain you all. You may choose the option that suits you. Your daughter would be completely under our rehabilitation program. When needed we may refer her for some other professional services? As I told you at the beginning low vision service is the beginning of the relationship. Not all services can be provided by one single professional. I have my own specialization about which we will talk later. But for now, you meet the receptionist. She would do the rest of formalities.

They ordered for telescope and a pair of pinhole contact lenses and thus we registered her in our low vision rehabilitation program.

COMPONENTS OF EFFECTIVE LOW VISION COUNSELING

An effective counseling is like a two-way street. It takes a cooperative effort by the person receiving the counseling and the counselor and it also takes a commitment to make some difficult changes, of course some times, in behavior or thinking pattern. The process of counseling is far too mysterious and complex to truly get a handle on all the nuances. But in low vision practice mostly, it is one-sided effort where the practitioner or his assistant spends time with the patient to explain the condition of his eyes and vision and motivates him to follow his advises regarding the use of gadgets and changes that the practitioner prescribes. This is the most important stage of the low vision practice as it determines the success of the practice. Therefore, it must be taken very seriously. There are some important elements that form the important components of the effective low vision patient counseling. These components are shown in **Flowchart 6.2**.

Preparation of the Session

Successful counseling requires preparation. However, in low vision practice if the practitioner himself counsels, he may not require to spend time on preparations as he has been in touch with the patient from the beginning, so he knows him and his medical history,

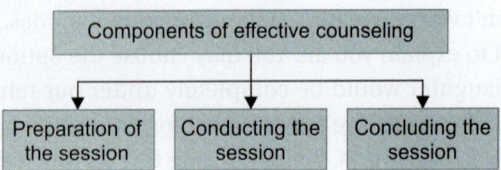

Flowchart 6.2: Components of effective low vision counseling.

understands his psychological condition, and can reasonably anticipate the expected behavioral response. In case the responsibility is delegated to someone else in the clinic, solid preparation is essential to effective counseling. The counselor should review all pertinent information. This includes the following:
- Patient medical history including his general and ocular health
- Impact of ocular condition on lifestyle
- Current visual status
- Patient's expectations and motivational factors
- The purpose of his visit
- Practitioner's instructions and recommendations
- Treatment plan and follow-ups

He can gather all the information from the patient's record file. Additionally, he may also take practitioner's feedback and his critical observations before starting the counseling session with the patient. Once these preparations are done, he can select the appropriate place and establish the right atmosphere to conduct the counseling session.

Conducting the Session

While conducting the counseling session, the low vision counselor should be flexible. Often counseling occurs spontaneously as counselors encounter the patient in his routine practice. The purpose is to guide effective counseling rather than mandate a series of rigid steps. However, while conducting counseling session he should address the following basic components:
- Setting up the context
- Briefing the results of the low vision examination
- Low vision prescription and its application
- Making necessary records, if any
- Use of gadgets and its effect on his function vision
- Commercial involved and payment plans
- Follow-ups needed
- Additional services needed

In the session opening, the counselor should state the purpose of the session and establish a client-centered setting. The best way to open a counseling session is to clearly state the purpose of the session. As he goes deeper, the aim should be to help the patient understand the prescription and future course of action. The counselor must be honest and fair in explaining the applications of the gadgets and must try and make effort to motivate to take decisions with sensible expectations.

Concluding the Session

Documenting the important point of discussion during counseling is always recommended as it serves as a reference points to the agreed points upon plan of action, patient's agreement, preferences, or problems. In order to conclude the session, the counselor should summarize the key points and ask the patient if he understands the plan and how does he think. The session may end up with positive patient's response or the patient may postpone the decision for future. In the second case, the counselor must schedule future meeting before terminating the session.

SELECT THE CORRECT ANSWER

1. All of the following are the objectives of low vision counseling except....
   a. To give the patient information on the current status of his visual condition
   b. To understand patient's readiness to accept the complete low vision rehabilitation program as a way of life
   c. To encourage and develop special abilities and right attitude toward low vision services and to help patients attend their immediate problems and also to equip them to meet future problems
   d. To discover the patient's visual concerns

2. All of the following are the traits of good low vision counselor except...
   a. Self-confidence
   b. A great speaker
   c. Flexibility and passion
   d. Multicultural competency

Chapter 6: Patient Counseling

3. How should low vision practitioner treat the patient who is not ready to listen to his advice?
    a. Disregard and the patient
    b. Take the fee and ask him to go
    c. Encourage the patient to educate himself and come back to him, if he wants to understand in details
    d. Discuss the importance of personal responsibility

4. When counseling patient to embrace low vision rehabilitation program as a way of life, which of the following approaches would be the best way to develop a patient's trust and build rapport?
    a. Demonstrate your commitment, be truthful, and uphold your integrity
    b. Include patient's family members in the conversation
    c. Include your assistant to support you in the conversation
    d. Confront the patient with targeted questions

Answers

| 1. d | 2. b | 3. c | 4. a |

SELF-PRACTICING QUESTIONS

1. How is patient's counseling different from patient's history taking?
2. Based upon the concept explained in the chapter write, how would you like to counsel a male patient, age 65 years, who has been diagnosed age-related macular degeneration (ARMD) for the first time and has been referred to low vision practice by an ophthalmologist?

CHAPTER 7

Visual Field Examination

Chapter Outline
- Objective of Visual Field Test
- Types of Visual Field Defects
- Tests for Visual Field Defects for Low Vision Patients

Visual field of an individual refers to the whole area that is seen while looking straight ahead when the eyes, head, and body are still. The peripheral visual field is the outer edges of the field. Normal monocular visual field extends up to 60° nasally, 60° superiorly, 70° inferiorly, and 100° temporarily as shown in **Figure 7.1**. Blindspot, the physiological scotoma exists at 15° degree temporally where the optic nerve leaves the eye.

The binocular visual field is the superimposition of the two monocular fields as shown in **Figure 7.2**.

OBJECTIVE OF VISUAL FIELD TEST

Visual field test in low vision patient is done with following objectives:
- To determine the magnification or minification
- To determine the need for prismatic lenses

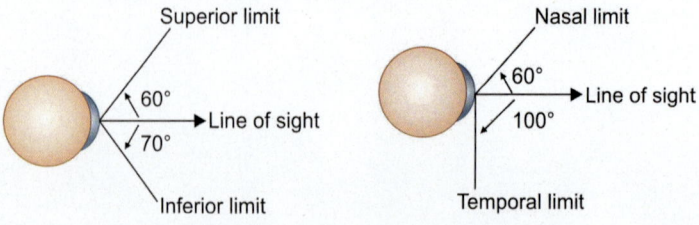

Fig. 7.1: Monocular visual field of an individual.

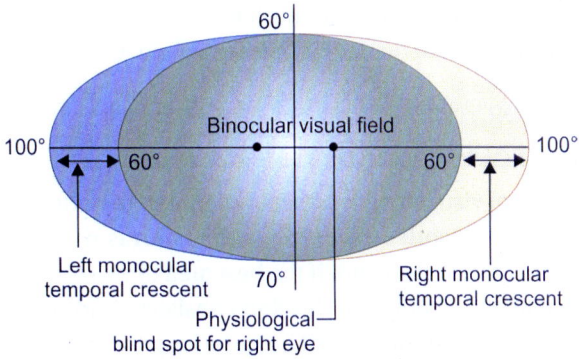

Fig. 7.2: Binocular visual field of an individual.

- To develop a full scope rehabilitation program for a patient
- To check eccentric fixation due to scotoma
- To determine eccentric viewing and fixation skills
- To record any apparent eccentric viewing angle.

TYPES OF VISUAL FIELD DEFECTS

A visual field defect is a loss of part of the normal field of vision. The lesion may be anywhere along the optic pathway from retina to occipital cortex. The visual field defect may be observed as:

- Central visual field defect is because of lesion in fovea or macula. Examples are an optic disk or nerve problem.
- Peripheral visual field defect may be anywhere along the visual pathways from the optic chiasm back.
- Scotoma is an area of partial diminished or entirely degenerated visual acuity that is surrounded by normal visual field. It may begin as a gradual enlargement of the blind spot and may pass unnoticed by the patient until quite large.
- Bitemporal hemianopia, the two halves lost are on the outside of each eye's peripheral vision.
- Homonymous hemianopia, the two halves lost are on the corresponding area of the visual field in both eyes, i.e., either the left or the right half of the visual field.
- Altitudinal hemianopia, the dividing line between visual loss and sight is horizontal, with visual loss either above or below the line.

- Quadrantanopia is an incomplete hemianopia referring to a quarter of the schematic "pie" of visual field loss.

TESTS FOR VISUAL FIELD DEFECTS FOR LOW VISION PATIENTS

The purpose of visual field tests is functional so that the information on visual field is collected before a decision is made about the prescription of low vision aid. If the best area of vision is known, it is easier to teach the patient to develop consistent and reliable visual input about the environment. The better a patient uses his vision without aid, the easier it will be to provide an optical aid that will work successfully. There are three different types of visual field tests as shown in **Flowchart 7.1** that are commonly used in low vision practice.

Amsler Grid Test

Amsler grid contains evenly spaced horizontal and vertical lines, making square boxes. Each square box is 5 mm square which subtends a visual angle of 1° on the retina when the chart is held at 30 cm distance. Thus, the test measures the central 10° from fixation spot, corresponding to central 10° of retina from the fovea.

Indications

The test should be applied in the following cases:
- When the patient visual acuity does not improve with pinhole
- When macula or optic nerve disease is suspected
- When patient's color vision is abnormal
- In all old patients.

Flowchart 7.1: Three visual field tests commonly used in low vision practice.

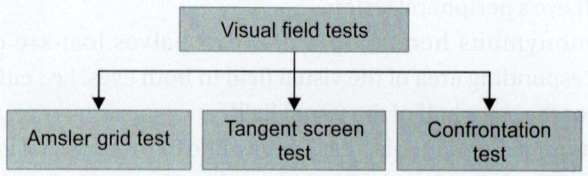

Objective

The test is valuable for determining the position and size of central scotomas. It was originally developed by Marc Amsler to allow patients to test their own central vision for early signs of macular degeneration, so that it may be treated sooner. The test is used to achieve following objectives:
- To determine the location and extent of central scotomas
- To determine the size of scotoma
- To detect metamorphopsia
- To develop a program for training in eccentric viewing that the instructor may use with the patient, i.e. direction in which the patient should view eccentrically.
- To determine the possible affectivity of the optical aid. If the patient can see the fixation spot with several squares around fixation spot, it can be anticipated that the magnification will work for the patient. Larger scotoma will inhibit the use of magnifier.
- To locate the best area of functional retina for prism image relocation.

Test Distance

The charts are made to be used at a distance of 28-30 cm, the usual distance for reading tests.

Room Lights

The chart must be clearly and evenly lighted as for a reading test.

Position of the Patient

The patient should be sitting on the chair with his refractive correction.

Precondition

Avoid all artificial mydriasis, as well as any ophthalmoscopy immediately before examination.

Test Charts

The Amsler grid charts are of various types:

Chapter 7: Visual Field Examination

Chart 1

The chart as shown in **Figure 7.3** is the standard chart, which must be used in every case and in many cases, it is sufficient.

Chart 2

This chart as shown in **Figure 7.4** is used for cases where central point is not seen. The diagonal lines help to fix the center of the square in spite of a central scotoma.

Chart 3

Figure 7.5 shows the standard chart again, but red on black, to be used in cases of color scotoma.

Chart 4

Figure 7.6 shows the chart with no lines, it reveals only the scotoma. There is no form to be disturbed. It consists of random dots and is used to differentiate scotoma from metamorphopsia.

Chart 5

Figure 7.7 shows the chart with parallel lines. It must be looked at horizontally and vertically. It shows metamorphopsia.

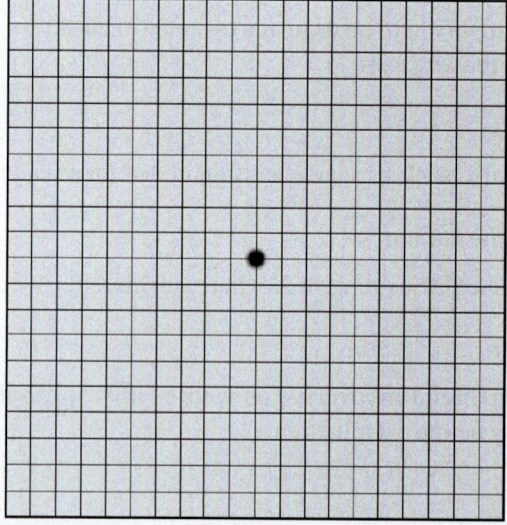

Fig. 7.3: Standard Amsler grid chart.

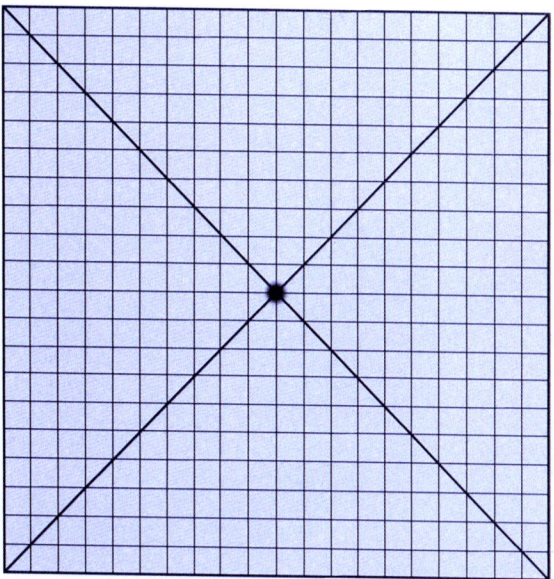

Fig. 7.4: Standard Amsler grid chart with diagonal lines.

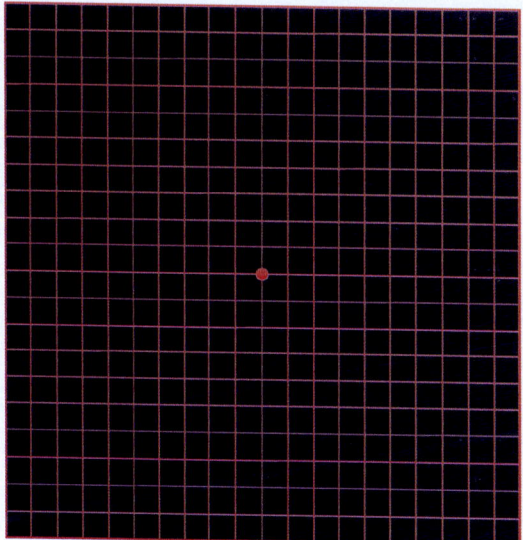

Fig. 7.5: Standard Amsler grid chart with red on black.

Fig. 7.6: Random dots Amsler chart.

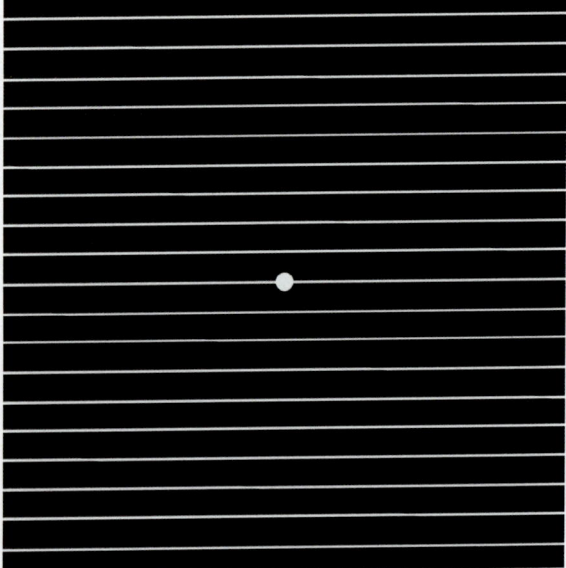

Fig. 7.7: Amsler chart with lines.

Fig. 7.8: Amsler chart with lines.

Chart 6

Figure 7.8 shows another chart for metamorphopsia, which allows a more minute examination of distribution along the reading lines.

Chart 7

Figure 7.9 shows the chart that allows more minute examination of the juxtacentral areas, where the rectangle with subdivided squares indicates the limits of the fovea.

Test Procedure

The patient must always keep his gaze fixed on the central point during the whole examinations with all charts and the practitioner must ceaselessly call the patient's attention to this. The sequence in which these tests are done varies from clinician to clinician.

Interpretation of Test Results

The grid indicates the position of scotomas and the areas of constricted field. **Table 7.1** shows the interpretation guideline for the areas of constricted field as discovered using Amsler grid test.

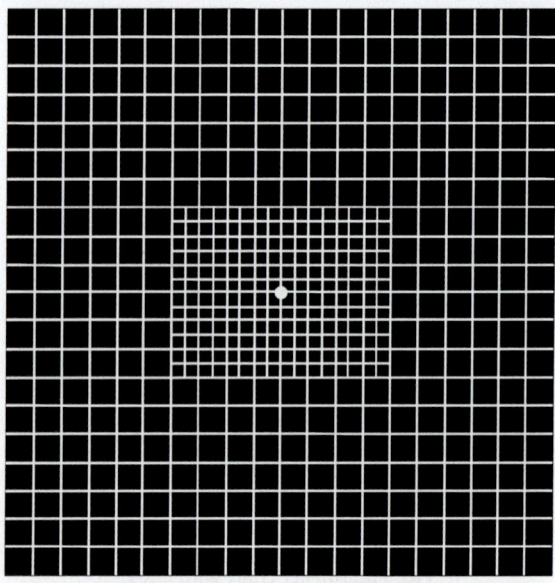

Fig. 7.9: Amsler grid chart for more minute examination.

Table 7.1: Amsler grid test results interpretation guideline.		
Location of scotoma	*Interpretation*	*Low vision management*
Fixation spot not seen	Fovea or macula lesion	Eccentric viewing technique
Fixation spot with some square not seen	Small loss of central visual field	Magnification may work
Scotoma to the right of fixation spot	Affects patient's reading ability as he is reading into the blind spot	Prism may be used to shift the image
Scotoma to the left of fixation spot	Difficulties in locating the beginning of next line	Typoscope may be used to drop down to next line
Large and absolute scotoma	Large central field defect	Optical aid may not work. CCTV may work

(CCTV: closed-circuit television)

Limitation of the Test

If the patient has already developed eccentric viewing, they will be able to fixate at the fixation spot regardless of the instruction and the patient may not see any defect on the grid.

Tangent Screen Test

Tangent screen **(Fig. 7.10)** measures the integrity of central 25–35° of field of vision. Blind spots in this area are most destructive to acuity and mobility and are often indicative of additional problem in the periphery. The patient sits on a chair and the test chart is placed at a distance of 1 m from the patient. The patient should be wearing his habitual distance correction lenses. If the patient is presbyopic, additional +1.00 D should be placed in front of his distance correction lenses when the chart is placed at 1 m distance. The patient should not be using his multifocal lenses. At first the test is done monocularly.

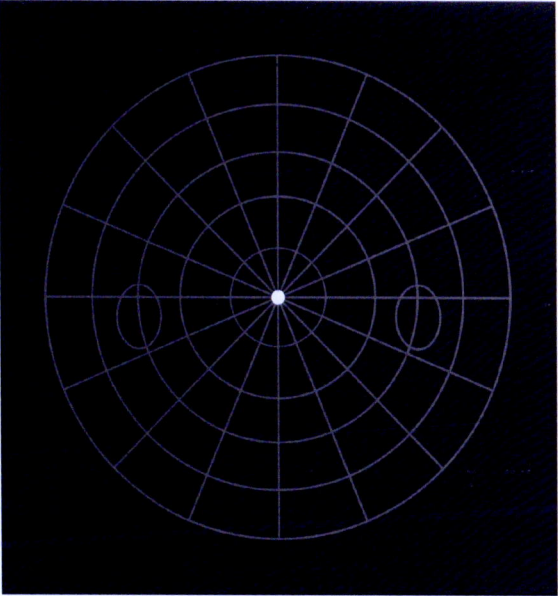

Fig. 7.10: Tangent screen.

The following steps are followed:
- Ask the patient to fixate at the central dot. If the patient is unable to fixate at the central dot, it implies central visual field loss and a cross-screen is used to help patient fixate at the central fixation dot.
- The examiner stands beside the test chart. He brings in a target from the sides and asks the patient to report when the target is seen.
- The nasal field represents temporal retina and temporal field represents nasal retina.
- The examiner should observe patient's posture and viewing technique during the test to get more meaningful interpretation of the test results.

Confrontation Test

With confrontation field assessment **(Fig. 7.11)**, we can obtain a rough peripheral field assessment without an expensive apparatus. Functionally, the loss of peripheral field inhibits the information processing abilities of the visual system as not enough information is taken at a time. To compensate for such defect, the patient must learn systematically to scan the environment to obtain meaningful information.

To do a confrontation field test, occlude one of the patient's eyes and have the patient fixate on your nose as you sit one-third of a meter from his eye. Slowly move a target, such as a penlight, in a semi-circular fashion from behind the patient's ear to in front of your nose and ask the patient to indicate when he first begins to see the light. Remember to keep the target about 13 inches or one-third of a meter from the patient's eye at all times. Make sure the patient continually stares at your nose and that the penlight is not aimed directly into his eye. Continue with the semi-circular areas around the perimeter of the patient's face until you are satisfied that the response has been accurate. If the patient has given no response to the target until it reached a point slightly inside your face line, the patient may have a restricted field of 15° or less. Other targets may include small puppets, toys, wiggling fingers or your hand, etc. Use your imagination, but keep the target size no bigger than about 10–20 mm.

The objective of all the visual field tests is to collect the information about best area of vision which will in turn help the examiner to train

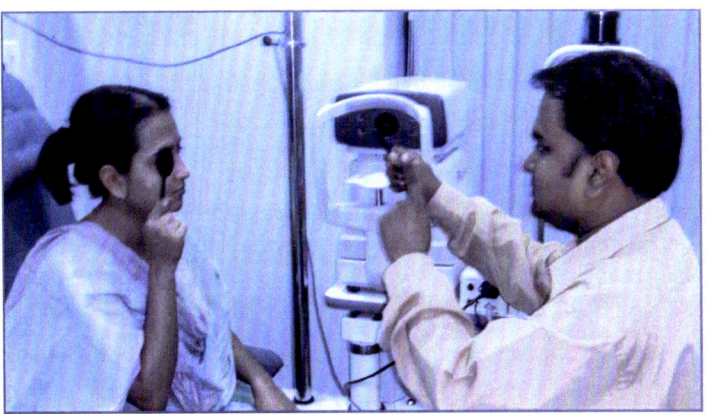

Fig. 7.11: An approximation of the visual field can be obtained with confrontation technique

Table 7.2: Ocular diseases associated with visual fields defects.

Ocular diseases	Visual field defects
ARMD	Central or paracentral scotoma with normal peripheral field
Retinitis pigmentosa	Loss of peripheral field of vision, leading to tunnel vision
Glaucoma	Reduced peripheral vision
Diabetic retinopathy	Corresponding visual field defects to the site of retinal ischemia, laser scars, and retinal detachment
Retinal detachment	Corresponding to the site of detachment
Optic atrophy	Central and paracentral visual field defects
Histoplasmosis	Central scotomas
Hemianopia	Visual field loss on the left or right side of the vertical midline.
Macular holes	Dense central scotoma

(ARMD: age-related macular degeneration)

the patient to use his residual vision more effectively. The better a patient uses his residual vision without aid, the better he will be able to perform with prescribed aids. Different ocular diseases are associated with different visual field defects which have been shown in **Table 7.2**.

Chapter 7: Visual Field Examination

SELECT THE CORRECT ANSWER

1. Which of the following is relevant in low vision examination regarding visual field defects?
   a. Visual field defects may have adverse effect on response to visual acuity test.
   b. Central field loss suggests the need for eccentric viewing training.
   c. Peripheral visual field loss suggests the need for orientation and mobility training.
   d. All of the above

2. Which of the following is not relevant as far as eccentric viewing technique is concerned?
   a. Eccentric viewing technique involves identifying an area of the retina that retains reasonable functionality and is as close to fovea as possible.
   b. Eccentric viewing technique involves improving the retinal functioning of the patient's eyes.
   c. If eccentric viewing is not consistent, the response to fixed optical magnification may vary resulting in variable responses and increased probability of frustration for examiner and patient alike.
   d. Not everyone with central vision loss will need to eccentrically fixate. It depends on the type and amount of scotoma(s).

3. Amsler grid tests suggest scotoma to the right of fixation spot, which of the following low vision management may work more effectively?
   a. Prism may be prescribed.
   b. Magnification may be used.
   c. Eccentric viewing technique may be suggested.
   d. Typoscopes may be used to block the right areas of objects.

Answers

1. d	2. b	3. a

SELF-PRACTICING QUESTION

1. What is the normal visual field test results? What can cause the visual field defects?

CHAPTER 8

Contrast Sensitivity and Glare Test

Chapter Outline

- Contrast Sensitivity
- Need for Contrast Sensitivity Test in Low Vision
- Method for Contrast Sensitivity Assessment
- Tests Charts for Contrast Sensitivity Test
- Glare Test

The vision is the function of partly on the use to which the eyes are put and the associated environment, partly on the efficiency of the visual system and partly on the individual's capacity to sustain effort. Lack of contrast between the object and its background and the glare often cause unpleasant visual experience. The impact of both can manifest significantly in low vision patient. Therefore, in low vision practice assessment of contrast sensitivity and light evaluation along with elimination of glare should be routinely performed when the patient's performance does not match the expected results.

CONTRAST SENSITIVITY

There are three distinct terms that need to be understood when we talk about contrast sensitivity test—contrast, contrast threshold, and contrast sensitivity.

Contrast is the relative ratio of the brightness of a target with respect to its background.

Contrast threshold is the minimum perceptible contrast that is critical to see the object.

Contrast sensitivity refers to the ability of the visual system to distinguish between an object and its background **(Fig. 8.1)**. It is

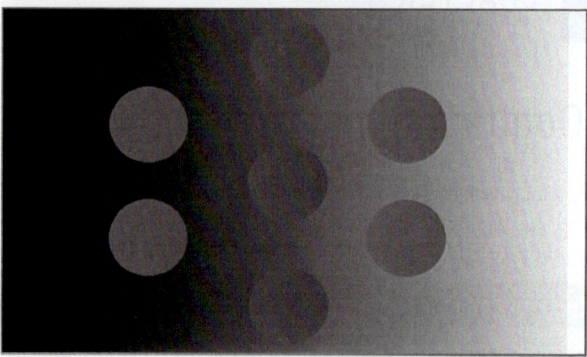

Fig. 8.1: Compare gray circle against a dark background vs. light background.

a critical component of functionally adequate vision and can be understood as reciprocal of contrast threshold.

Contrast sensitivity tests measure the ability of the visual system to distinguish between an object and its background. Contrast sensitivity determines the lowest contrast level which can be detected by a patient for a given size of the object. Contrast sensitivity is a detection task, much like auditory testing as opposed to an identification task like visual acuity. It is purely a qualitative test, and tests the functional vision, i.e., how well an individual sees everyday visual objects or scenes. Contrast sensitivity testing provides a comprehensive assessment of everyday vision. It only measures small changes or losses in vision. The results of contrast sensitivity tests will better predict everyday visual performance, as everyday life is full of high and low contrast situations.

Unlike a visual acuity of 20/20, there is no single magic value or a set of values that describe the contrast sensitivity of a normal patient. The best course of action for the clinician is to establish a baseline contrast sensitivity measurement for each patient at their initial visit. Contrast sensitivity is drastically reduced in many diseases such as corneal opacities, cataract, optic nerve atrophy, and retinal degeneration. The test therefore can be a useful tool to detect ocular disease at the early stage and also monitor the condition. Aging also affects contrast sensitivity. Older people often find it difficult to see clearly in low contrast situation.

Chapter 8: Contrast Sensitivity and Glare Test

NEED FOR CONTRAST SENSITIVE TEST IN LOW VISION

Even though visual acuity testing is so deeply ingrained in the clinical eye care of our patients, it tells very little about the patient's visual system. Contrast sensitivity test is a useful tool in the early detection of various diseases as well as in the determination of any complications arising from a routine procedure. Two personnel with the same Snellen acuity can function differently which may be predicted with the contrast sensitivity test. It is important to understand that blur vision is not the same as poor contrast.

In general, a poor contrast indicates that the clinician should give more attention to glare control, contrast of viewing materials, and illuminations. These factors are often more important than magnification. A patient may be doing poorly with 3× magnification, but simply by adding a halogen light to the 3× magnifier, optimum visual functioning can be achieved and without such light, it may take 5× magnification to achieve the same visual functioning.

A low contrast curve suggests that the patient may need double or triple the power of magnification that would have been calculated on the basis of the reciprocal of the acuity. In addition, there is a threshold limit below which one can predict the negligible response to the magnification. It is therefore always recommended to perform the contrast sensitivity test on all patients at their initial visit.

A notable difference between high contrast and low contrast acuity may alert the practitioner to monitor the visual system more closely. Many researchers prefer to prescribe the monocular aid with eye with better contrast sensitivity than better visual acuity.

METHODS FOR CONTRAST SENSITIVITY ASSESSMENT

Contrast sensitivity is assessed with the best correction in place and is tested by viewing the targets of varying contrasts and sizes (spatial frequency) to relate how well a person functions visually to see every day object. Pupil should be in their natural (undilated) state. Various charts are available for the purpose and the procedure for the respective chart has to be followed. It is always recommended to use two different methods and investigate changes in the shape of the curve of the test results under different viewing conditions. Proceed monocularly with the better eye previously determined by visual acuity and Amsler grid test, and then the fellow eye. The lowest point (threshold) at which the grating orientation can be identified accurately is determined. The results are presented on a chart that shows the threshold for a number of different grating spacing. To complete the test, compare these findings with the binocular responses, starting at the level of the best monocular answer. The binocular response is more significant than the either eye alone.

TESTS CHARTS FOR CONTRAST SENSITIVITY TEST

Several contrast tests charts are available—the key difference is the target type. They are as described below.

Sine-Wave Contrast Test

Sine-wave gratings are special test pattern for contrast sensitivity testing. Sine-wave grating contrast sensitivity testing **(Fig. 8.2)** uses varying sizes and contrast of gray bars set up in circular pattern to test individual's ability to detect different gratings to identify the individual's visual contrast threshold. The handheld model is used to check contrast sensitivity for near at a distance of 1 m and wall mounted chart is used for distance at 3 m. This chart is printed with circular patches of sine wave gratings, which decreases in contrast from left to right and increases in spatial frequency from top to bottom.

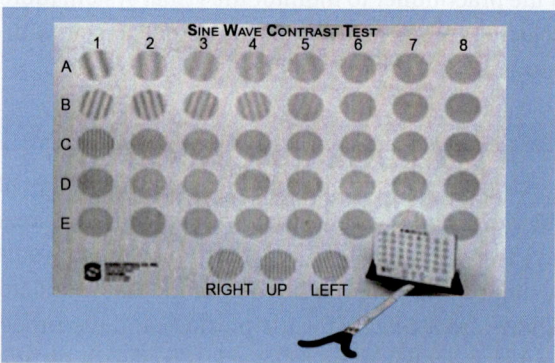

Fig. 8.2: Sine-wave contrast test chart.

The gratings are either vertical or tilted at 10° to the left or right of vertical. It is assumed if a patient can detect gratings, he will be able to describe its orientation whether left, right, or vertical. There are four possible responses: "Left," "right," "up," or "blank." The chart should be uniformly illuminated while testing. Starting with row A, ask the patient to identify the orientations of the grating patches moving from left to right. Use the graphical record sheet to record the number of the last patch correctly identified. Repeat the procedure for row B to E.

Low Contrast Letter Test

Letter chart determines the contrast required to read the letter by altering the contrast of the chart. For example, two charts are supplied printed with different sequence of letters, together with instructions for use and a scoring pad. Pelli-Robson chart **(Fig. 8.3)** uses the letter of the same size corresponding to 0.03 logMar at the test distance of 1 m. Letters of fixed size are used with reducing contrast to provide quick means of assessing patient's contrast sensitivity threshold. The Regan chart has different size letters. It reduces the contrast level of standard Snellen type letter acuity chart resulting in several charts.

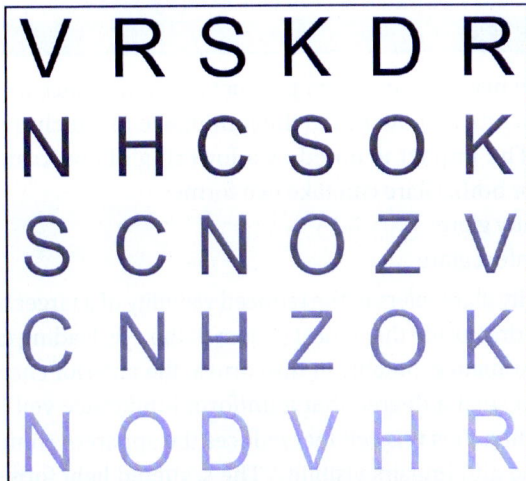

Fig. 8.3: Pelli-Robson chart.

Chapter 8: Contrast Sensitivity and Glare Test

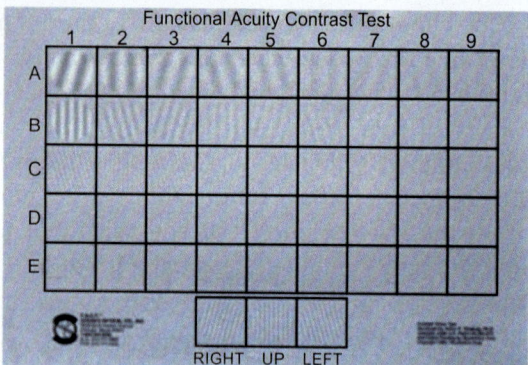

Fig. 8.4: Functional acuity contrast test chart.

Functional Acuity Contrast Test

Functional acuity contrast test (FACT) chart **(Fig. 8.4)** developed by Dr. Arthur P. Ginsburg uses sine-wave grating procedure. The chart tests five spatial frequencies (sizes) and nine levels of contrast. The patient determines the last grating seen for each row (A, B, C, D, and E) and reports the orientation of the gratings right, up, or left. The last correct grating seen for each spatial frequency is plotted on a contrast sensitivity curve.

GLARE TEST

Glare is the negative sensation produced by luminance in the visual field that is much greater than the luminance to which the eyes are adapted. The impact is noted as a lowering of contrast, reduced visibility, or both. Glare can take two forms:
1. Disability glare
2. Discomfort glare

Disability glare refers to the reduced visibility of a target because of light scattering inside the optical system of the eye, leading to reduced visual performance, notably in the cornea, the anterior chamber, and the lens, to such a degree that a uniform luminance veil is created over the retina. It is this veil that reduces the apparent contrast in the visual scene and impairs visibility. The scattered light forms a veil of luminance, which reduces the contrast and thus the visibility of the target. Disability glare may be caused by cataracts, keratoconus, corneal edema, vitreous opacities, etc.

Discomfort glare is a sensation of discomfort or even pain caused by excessive luminance in the field of view. Discomfort glare usually occurs when overall illumination is too bright or varies in luminosity within the visual field. The size and position of the source or sources relative to the viewing direction determine the impact of discomfort glare.

Glare can be caused by high-intensity light sources that are out of the field of vision. When the sun is directly overhead, the wearing of a cap serves to provide the necessary screening. There are two types of glare in particular:
1. Direct glare
2. Indirect glare

Direct glare is caused by high luminance from a light source present in the field of view. Reflected glare results from the reflection of light from a polished surface within the field of view. For instance, the reflection of the sun on a mirror can cause discomfort.

Though the clinical measurement of discomfort glare is difficult as no test is commercially available, in low vision rehabilitation, discomfort glare can be avoided by changing the light's brightness or position in the visual environment. However, low vision practise is more concerned with the disability glare that arises because of light scatter within the ocular media. Disability glare can be determined by measuring contrast sensitivity or visual acuity after placing a glare source in the periphery of the patient's visual field. The drop in the score may be considered an effect of glare. When there is a reduction in image quality because of glare, overall changes in illumination may be effective in enhancing the visual performance, either by increasing or decreasing the illumination level.

SELECT THE CORRECT ANSWER

1. Contrast sensitivity test is the measure of ...
    a. The eye sensitivity to light
    b. Ability of the eye to detect the luminance contrast
    c. The visual acuity
    d. The motion sensitivity

2. The following statements regarding the role of the contrast sensitivity testing are true, except...
   a. Contrast sensitivity testing is useful in detecting diseases in patients with normal and near normal acuity
   b. Loss of contrast sensitivity usually occurs in pattern specific to different ocular pathologies
   c. Contrast sensitivity is routinely measured in general eye care practice to diagnose and monitor ocular diseases.
   d. The VISTECH chart is an example of contrast sensitivity test using sine-wave grating

3. Contrast sensitivity test helps practitioner determine the need for which of the following?
   a. Increased illumination
   b. Magnification
   c. Orientation and training
   d. Prism lenses

4. Which of the following factors is associated with reduction in contrast sensitivity?
   a. Aging
   b. Cataract
   c. Refractive surgery
   d. All of the above

Answers			
1. b	2. c	3. a	4. d

SELF-PRACTICING QUESTION

1. How does the results of contrast sensitivity test help in low vision patient rehabilitation?

CHAPTER 9

Common Causes of Low Vision

Chapter Outline

- Achromatopsia
- Age Related Macular Degeneration
- Diabetic Retinopathy
- Toxoplasmosis
- Albinism
- Retinitis Pigmentosa
- Histoplasmosis
- Stargardt's Diseases
- Aniridia
- Glaucoma
- Nystagmus
- Optic Atrophy
- Coloboma
- Cataract
- Retinal Detachment
- Keratoconus
- Hemianopia

The low vision practitioners must be familiar with signs, symptoms, and the visual disturbances associated with various ocular diseases. Different ocular diseases cause different visual disturbances and accordingly their management has to be decided. The most common causes of low vision are as follows:

ACHROMATOPSIA

Condition

Total color blindness.

Area Affected

Retina (cone malformation).

Visual Defects

- Decreased visual acuity to about 20/200
- Inability to discriminate colors
- Near vision is less affected than distance
- Extreme photophobia
- Nystagmus
- Visual fields are normal.

Low Vision Aids

- Dim illumination
- Sunglasses
- Filters
- Visors.

AGE-RELATED MACULAR DEGENERATION

Condition

The macula in the retina degenerates, causing a gradual or sudden loss of vision **(Fig. 9.1)**.

Area Affected

Macula.

Visual Defects

- Fuzzy and decreased vision
- Metamorphopsia, i.e., patient sees distortions. A straight line appears wavy.
- Poor central vision but good side vision **(Fig. 9.1)**.
- Blind spots, i.e., small areas of vision loss. The objects are seen when they fall on peripheral retina and disappeared when they fall within the blind spots, i.e., central scotomas.
- Photophobia

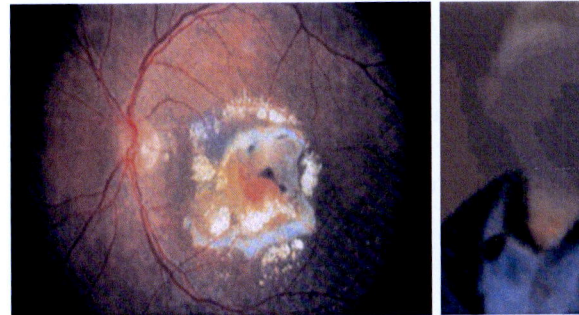

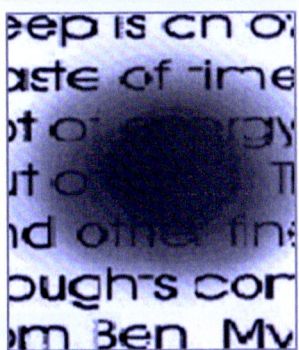

Fig. 9.1: Macular degeneration.

- Comparatively better vision at night
- Color perception is poor as highest concentration of cone cells are in the macula.
- Depth perception is impaired.

Low Vision Aids

- Good lighting. Use extra light from adjustable lamp for close work.
- Use strong colors and color contrasts.
- Magnifiers are useful with illuminations.
- Vision rehabilitation is required to promote eccentric viewing. Try looking at the objects from the side of eyes, not directly at them.
- Sit close to the television.
- Monocular telescopes may be used in some cases to locate street signs and spotting general environmental clues.

DIABETIC RETINOPATHY

Condition

Diabetic retinopathy is the name given to the changes in the retina of the eye which can occur over time in people who have diabetes. The walls of the blood vessels start to break, leaking blood around them **(Fig. 9.2)**.

Area Affected

Retina.

Visual Defects

- Gradually decreased visual acuity
- Fluctuating vision
- Loss of color vision or visual field
- Inability to accommodate
- Floaters.

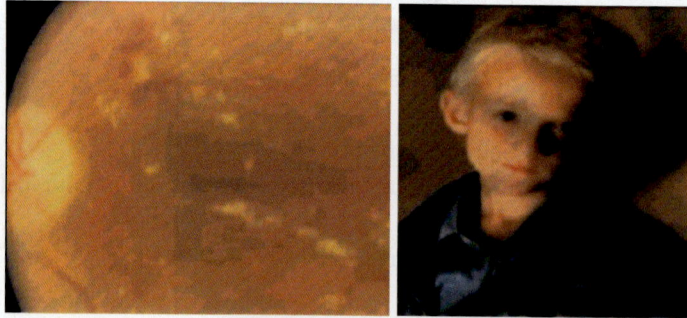
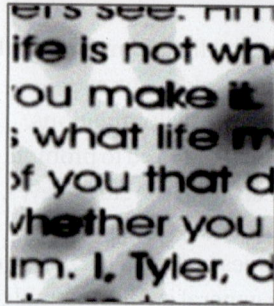

Fig. 9.2: Effect of diabetic retinopathy.

Low Vision Aids

- Various illumination control aids
- Use caps or visors in sun
- For close work try direct light from an adjustable lamp
- Visual rehabilitation like avoiding glare, light shining directly into the eyes or reflecting back off a shiny surface.

TOXOPLASMOSIS

Condition

Severe intraocular infection, may be congenital or acquired.

Area Affected

Retina, especially macular lesions.

Visual Defects

- Loss in visual fields corresponding to location of lesions
- Squint
- Decreased visual acuity if macula is affected
- Floaters.

Low Vision Aids

Usually good response to magnifier.

ALBINISM

Condition

Total or partial loss of pigments in the eye, skin, or hair characterized by light colored iris, eyebrows, and platinum-blonde hair **(Fig. 9.3)**.

Area Affected

Abnormal development of retina, macula underdeveloped, and abnormal connection between the eye and brain.

Visual Defects

- Decreased visual acuity to 20/200 to 20/70.
- Distance vision is more affected than near.

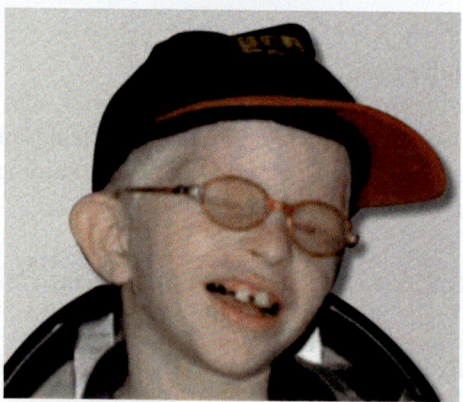

Fig. 9.3: Albinism.

- Painful photophobia.
- Nystagmus, irregular rapid movement of eyes.
- High refractive error with severe astigmatism. When refractive error is corrected, they do not show expected increase in acuity because macula is not fully developed.
- Color vision is normal.
- Visual fields are normal or slightly reduced.

Low Vision Aids

- Visors or caps
- Dim illumination
- Colored or pinhole type contact lens to prevent light passing through iris
- Dense sunglasses
- Absorptive lenses
- Telescope for distance vision
- For reading work, place light over shoulder rather than in front.

RETINITIS PIGMENTOSA

Condition

Retinal pigmentary degeneration. Rods of retina are slowly destroyed (Fig. 9.4).

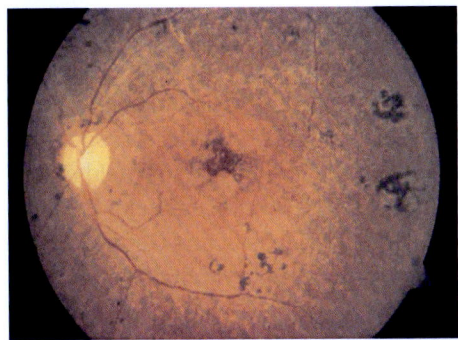
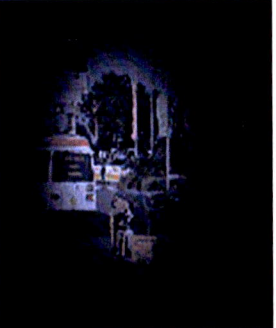
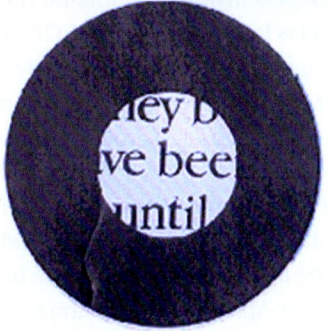

Fig. 9.4: Retinitis pigmentosa.

Area Affected

Retina.

Visual Defects

- Difficulty in seeing at night or in poor illumination leading to night blindness
- Decreased visual acuity
- Photophobia
- Loss of peripheral field of vision, leading to tunnel vision
- Poor contrast sensitivity
- In later stage, central vision may be affected due to macular damage
- Difficulty to adapt in changing illumination.

Low Vision Aids

- *Management of peripheral field of vision:* Reverse Galilean telescope may be used but it reduces the visual acuity. Fresnel prisms can be successfully applied in case of decreased visual acuity. Placement of base out on the temporal visual field makes objects appear more toward the center of visual field. Besides, Door eye, Inwave retinitis pigmentosa lenses, and Gottlieb visual field awareness systems are also visual field expanders.
- *Management of night blindness:* Night blindness may be dealt with increasing light levels inside and outside home. In some cases, where night travel is frequent NIGHTSCOPES may be employed.
- *Management of light adaptation:* Amber filters of varying density or corning color protect filter (CPF) lenses may help. Hats and visors are often helpful and wrap around sunwear with side shields are helpful tools.
- *Management of decreased central vision with loss of peripheral vision:* High contrast letters, closed-circuit television (CCTV), or magnifiers may be applied on case-to-case basis.
- *Vision rehabilitation:* Apart from low vision aid, some rehabilitation is also needed. For example, changes in walking speed and scanning the environment, introduction of long cane, etc.

HISTOPLASMOSIS

Condition
Intraocular fungal infection.

Area Affected
Macula or peripheral retina.

Visual Defects
The effect on vision depends on the location and extent of lesions, if macula is affected:
- Both distance vision and near vision acuity reduce
- Central scotomas
- Deficient color vision
- Decreased central visual acuity

- Words, lines, or poles may appear wavy or distorted
- Decreased depth perception
- Photostress and photophobia
- "Come and go" vision.

Low Vision Aids

If one eye is affected, safety eye wear is advised to protect the remaining vision in the good eye. If both the eyes are visually impaired:
- High power reading eye wear
- Magnifiers
- CCTV
- Sun filters
- Eccentric viewing.

STARGARDT DISEASES

Condition

Stargardt diseases are recessive progressive retinal dystrophy of the central retina and develop before the age of 20 years. They cause gradual deterioration of retina's cone receptor cells.

Area Affected

Macula.

Visual Defects

- Blurred vision, not correctable with traditional glasses or contact lenses
- Photostress
- Progressive loss of central vision
- Peripheral vision is not affected
- Diminished ability to perceive colors
- Missing areas of central vision.

Low Vision Aids

Low vision aids are recommended to utilize the peripheral vision and remaining central vision. Lamps and large prints may be good trial. Magnifiers and telescopes also work in certain cases.

ANIRIDIA

Condition
Failure of the iris to develop fully so that the iris is partially or almost completely absent. It is a congenital defect and usually affects both eyes. The general appearance is that of an extremely large pupil.

Area Affected
Iris.

Visual Defects
- Extreme photophobia
- Decreased visual acuity
- Nystagmus
- Constriction of visual field (tunnel vision) may be present.

Low Vision Aids
- Dim illumination
- Sunglasses
- Pinhole contact lenses
- Optical aids
- Caps or visors.

GLAUCOMA (FIG. 9.5)

Condition
Aqueous humor does not drain normally and excessive pressure is built within the eye, resulting in damage to the optic nerve. It is often known as the "sneak thief of sight."

Area Affected
Optic nerve is damaged.

Visual Defects
- Blurred vision which is gradual
- Haloes around the light

Chapter 9: Common Causes of Low Vision

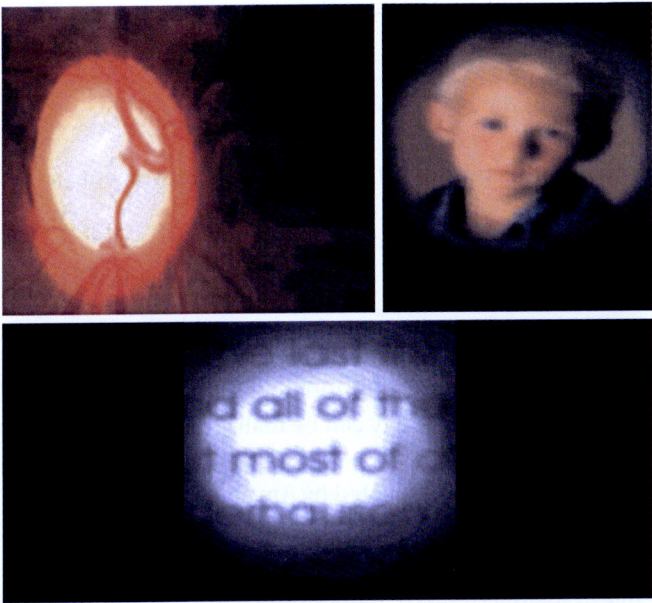

Fig. 9.5: Glaucoma.

- Reduced peripheral vision
- Photophobia.

Low Vision Aids

- Magnifiers depending upon the extent of visual field loss
- CCTV
- CPF lens to reduce glare.
- Prisms or mirror system may stimulate peripheral awareness.

NYSTAGMUS

Condition

Involuntary rhythmic shaking or wobbling of the eyes. Nystagmus may be seen very early in the life or may be acquired later also. Early nystagmus is usually the side effect of vision loss due to different eye diseases. In later stage, nystagmus may be acquired due to neurological dysfunction.

Area Affected

Neurological disorder.

Visual Defects

- Visual acuity is related to the amplitude of movement.
- Fluctuating vision
- Impairment of binocular vision
- Depth perception may be affected indirectly in some cases.

Low Vision Aids

- Better illumination and appropriate refractive correction
- Improvement in the acuity can be realized if the rate or extent of eye movement is reduced.
- Prism base out or as indicated by Amsler grid test.
- Spectacle magnifier for near
- Contact lens telescope
- Since nystagmus tends to reduce on accommodation, a binocular unit is preferable.

OPTIC ATROPHY

Condition

Degeneration of some or most of the optic nerve fibers. Many diseases or disorders can lead to optic atrophy. The nerve becomes totally pale white.

Area Affected

Optic nerve.

Visual Defects

- Permanent visual impairment
- Blurred vision
- Poor constriction of pupil in light
- Color vision deficits may be evident at the early stage
- Contrast discrimination may become difficult in early stage

- A general decrease of sensitivity in all visual fields
- Congenital optic atrophy in both eyes may lead to nystagmus.

Low Vision Aids

The following aids may be tried till optic atrophy is not complete:
- High illumination
- Enlarged print with high contrast
- Magnifiers may be useful in some cases
- Comprehensive visual rehabilitation is needed.

COLOBOMA

Condition

Coloboma is a congenital condition which describes a situation where the patient has a portion of the structure of the eye lacking. In colobomatous eye, the pupil looks like a tear-drop shape. It is generally bilateral.

Area Affected

The gap can occur either in the eyelid, iris, lens, choroid or optic disk, or all.

Visual Defects

- Decreased visual acuity **(Fig. 9.6)**
- Nystagmus and strabismus
- Photophobia
- Loss of visual fields **(Fig. 9.6)**
- Glare problem

Low Vision Aids

- Sunglasses for glare problem
- If pupil is cosmetically unattractive, the patient may be fitted with a cosmetic contact lens to make the pupil look normal.

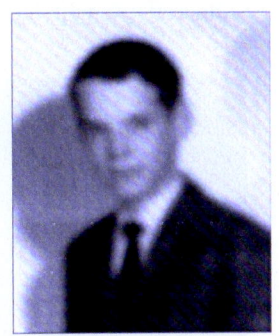

Fig. 9.6: Decreased visual acuity and visual field.

- Magnification for distance and near vision
- Nonoptical aids should be demonstrated.

CATARACT

Condition

Clouding or opacification of lens inside the eye, implying less light can get through to the retina and vision becomes hazy and inconsistent (**Fig. 9.7**).

Area Affected

Crystalline lens.

Visual Defects

- Blurred vision
- Nystagmus may be present in congenital cataract
- Serious glare problem and difficulty in bright light
- Seeing double if the clouding is in one eye
- If the patient wears glasses, he may constantly feel that they are scratched or need cleaning
- Visual fields are usually normal. There may be some reduction in the peripheral vision
- Development of the squint due to lack of visual stimulation of the affected eye, which results in amblyopia.

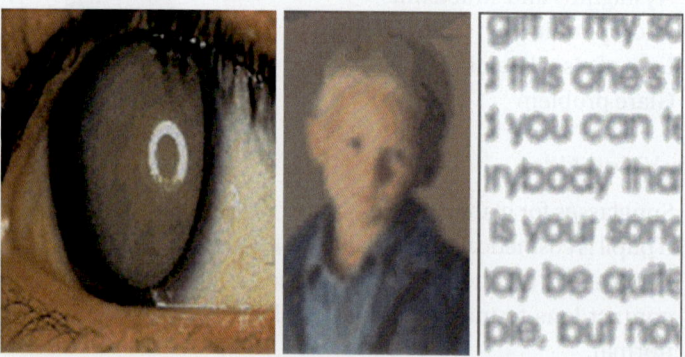

Fig. 9.7: Lens clouding and hazy vision.

Low Vision Aids

For the patients with cataracts, following options may be useful:
- For close work, use direct light from an adjustable lamp
- Use sunglasses and visors on sunny days
- Stand magnifier for near work
- Amber, red-brown, yellow-orange filters are useful.

A cataract is a disorder that can lead to severe visual impairment. However, successful lens removal usually results in complete visual recovery.

RETINAL DETACHMENT

Condition

Retina is separated from its supporting structures and receives no nourishment. The detached portion of the retina atrophies and a blind area develops in the field of vision corresponding to the area of detachment.

Area Affected

Retina.

Visual Defects

- Appearance of flashing lights
- If macula is involved, visual acuity may be decreased or lost
- Micropsia, i.e., objects appearing smaller when viewed with the affected eye
- Color vision may be impaired
- Loss of visual field
- Photophobia and glare.

Low Vision Aids

- High illumination.
- Photophobia and glare can be eliminated with tints, filters, or CPF lens.
- Magnification devices for distance and near may be helpful.
- Nonoptical aids should be demonstrated.

KERATOCONUS

Condition

Keratoconus is a bilateral, noninflammatory, progressive ectasia of the cornea characterized by thinning and steepening of the cornea. The cone-like protrusion produces progressive decrease in vision due to irregular myopic astigmatism **(Fig. 9.8)**.

Area Affected

Cornea.

Visual Defects

- Progressive decrease in visual acuity.
- No definite visual field defect but general distortion of field is noted.
- Starbursts around the objects.
- Monocular diplopia may occur as the disorder progresses.

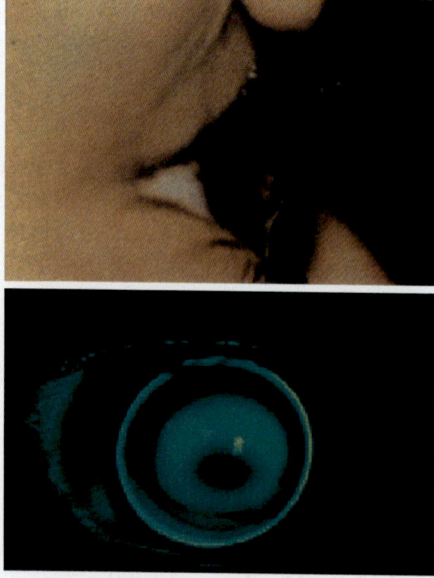

Fig. 9.8: Keratoconus.

Low Vision Aids

- Rigid gas permeable (RGP) lenses.
- A combination of piggyback lens system in case of RGP lens intolerance.
- Pinhole lens may be necessary to prevent "ghost image."
- Corning color protect filter (CPF), tinted, or filter lenses are helpful to avoid glare and photophobia.
- Some response to magnification at distance and near with more success with closed-circuit television (CCTV) at near.

Keratoconus manifests in adolescent years and can progress slowly, stabilizing during middle age or can advance rapidly requiring keratoplasty.

HEMIANOPIA

Condition
Hemianopia is the partial blindness or a loss of sight in half of the visual field **(Fig. 9.9)**.

Area Affected
Hemianopia is caused by brain damage, rather than a problem with the eyes.

Visual Defects
- Loss of half of the visual field in one or both eyes
- Dimmed and distorted sight

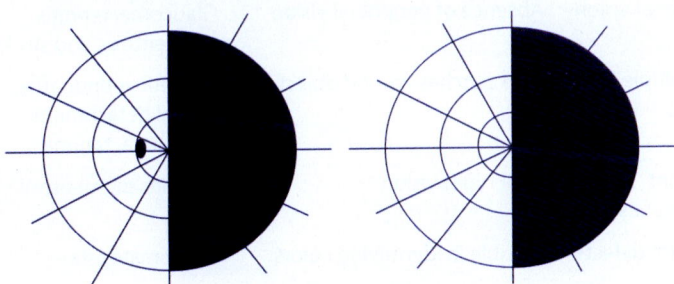

Fig. 9.9: Homonymous hemianopia.

- Difficulty understanding what is being seen
- Poor night vision
- Moving the body or head away from the affected side.

Low Vision Aids

- Inwave field expanding lenses
- Mirror system
- Prism lenses
- Typoscopes for reading.

Table 9.1 summarizes the common visual symptoms of low vision patients that are commonly observed in different ocular conditions.

Table 9.1: Visual symptoms of low vision patients.

Visual symptoms	Interpretation	Causes
Blur vision	Objects not in focus	ARMD, corneal disease, cataract, diabetic retinopathy
Poor contrast and glare effect	Difficult to discriminate the object from its background and intolerance to light	Glaucoma, cataract, corneal disease, and albinism
Distortion	Objects appeared deformed, wavy	ARMD, diabetic retinopathy, retinal detachment
Central visual field loss	Hazy patch in the center of the object	Macular degeneration and optic atrophy
Tunnel vision	Absence of peripheral vision	Glaucoma, retinitis pigmentosa, and stroke
Multiple field loss	Dark patches around objects	Diabetic retinopathy, retinal detachment, glaucoma, trauma
Night blindness	Poor night vision	Retinitis pigmentosa
Color defects	Trouble in identifying colors	Achromatopsia

(ARMD: age-related macular degeneration)

Chapter 9: Common Causes of Low Vision

SELECT THE CORRECT ANSWER

1. Achromatopsia is characterized by….
   a. It is a hereditary condition
   b. Absence of color discrimination
   c. Visual acuity is reduced but visual field is usually intact
   d. All of the above

2. Which of the following is true regarding ARMD?
   a. Central or paracentral visual field loss
   b. Peripheral visual field loss
   c. Sectoral visual field loss
   d. Temporal visual field loss

3. Which of the following ocular disorder would demonstrate nystagmus, photophobia, decreased acuity, and iris trans-illumination?
   a. Achromatopsia
   b. Keratoconus
   c. Albinism
   d. Toxoplasmosis

4. A patient has bitemporal hemianopia, the direction of the base of prism in spectacle lens should be…
   a. Nasal
   b. Temporal
   c. Inferior
   d. Superior

5. Which of the following is the first symptom is most commonly noticed in patient with retinitis pigmentosa?
   a. Night blindness
   b. Constriction of visual field
   c. Delay in dark and light adaptation speed
   d. Decreased color sensitivity

6. The appearance of flashing lights accompanied by sharp, stabbing pain in the eye are significant indication of…..
   a. Recent or impending retinal detachment
   b. Recent onset of macular degeneration
   c. Toxoplasmosis
   d. Histoplasmosis

7. Which of the following condition is associated with partial or complete absence of iris?
   a. Albinism
   b. Aniridia
   c. Uveitis
   d. Polycoria

8. Which of the following condition is the result of fungus infection?
   a. Toxoplasmosis
   b. Histoplasmosis
   c. Endophthalmitis
   d. All of the above

Answers			
1. d	2. a	3. c	4. b
5. a	6. a	7. b	8. b

SELF-PRACTICING QUESTIONS

1. Glaucoma is considered to be one of the most challenging pathology in terms of low vision management. Explain in detail.
2. Describe the common visual symptoms of low vision patients that are commonly observed in different ocular conditions commonly.

CHAPTER 10

Magnifications

Chapter Outline

- Relative Size Magnification
- Relative-distance Magnification
- Angular Magnification
- Projection Magnification
- Power of Magnification
- Predicting Magnification Required

Magnification is a method of increasing the size of the retinal image so that enough of the retina is stimulated to send an impulse through the optic nerve to the brain allowing an object to be perceived. The amount of magnification needed for a patient is determined only after the distance refractive error has been corrected. There are four ways of creating the magnification which are described below.

RELATIVE SIZE MAGNIFICATION

In relative size magnification **(Fig. 10.1)**, the actual size of the object is increased. As the size of the object is doubled, the retinal image size increases. Two examples are large print textbooks or the use of a felt tip pen instead of a micro tip pen for writing. Sometimes this method of providing magnification is more acceptable to an individual, especially for reading because it allows a normal reading distance.

$$\text{Magnification} = \frac{\text{New object size}}{\text{Old object size}}$$

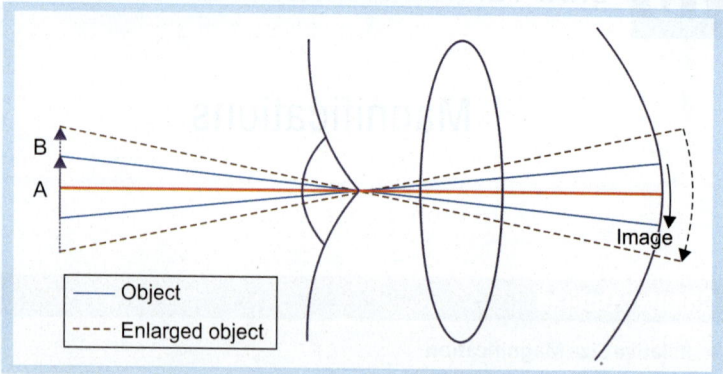

Fig. 10.1: Relative-size magnification increases the size of the retinal image by enlarging the actual size of the object.

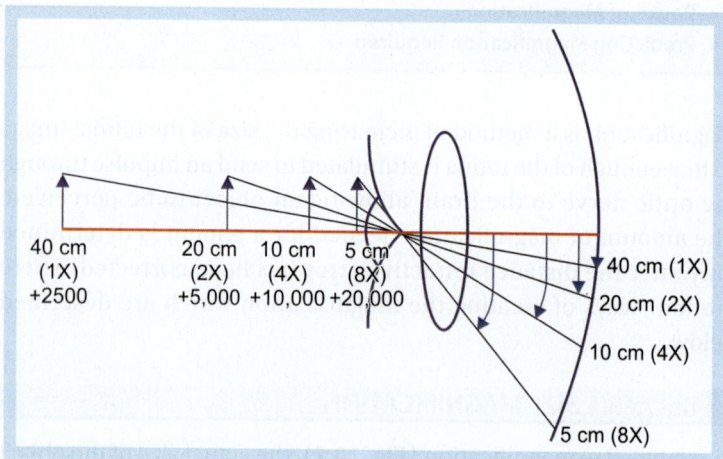

Fig. 10.2: In relative-distance magnification, the image enlarges proportionately as the object is brought closer to the eye.

RELATIVE-DISTANCE MAGNIFICATION

Relative-distance magnification, also known as approach magnification **(Fig. 10.2)**, simply means that as an object is brought closer to the eye, the retinal image becomes larger. The relationship is such that as an object is brought to one-half its present distance, the retinal image doubles. We must arbitrarily assign some distance as being a reference point so that it can be said that something is twice as big as something else.

Let us assume 40 cm as the reference distance. Thus, in the **Figure 10.2**, 1 × is the image size of an object held at 40 cm in front of the eye. When the object is brought to 20 cm, the magnification is 2×, at 10 cm, it is 4×, and at 5 cm, it is 8×, and so on. The enlargement occurs without the use of microscopic lens. The object at 40 cm will have light rays entering the eye with a divergence of –2.50 D (100/40 cm = –2.50 D). To get this enlarged image focused on the retina, the eye must accommodate +2.50 D, or a +2.50 D bifocal lens must be provided, or the patient must have –2.50 D of myopia, when the object is at 20 cm in front of the eye, the magnification is 2×, i.e., the retinal image of the object is twice as large as that of the retinal image of the object when the object was at 40 cm. Also, +5.00 D (100/20 = 5) lens, 5.00 D of accommodation, or 5.00 D myopia are needed to give a clear or focused image.

$$\text{Magnification} = \frac{\text{Old object distance}}{\text{New object distance}}$$

Two **Tables 10.1 and 10.2** show the distance magnification and lens power scheme at a reference distance of 40 cms and 25 cms respectively.

It can be seen that 4× magnification can be caused by a 16.00 D lens and also by 10.00 D lens depending upon the distance at which

Table 10.1: Magnification and lens power scheme at a reference distance of 40 cm.		
Distance of object (in cm)	Magnification	Lens needed
40	1×	2.50 D
20	2×	5.00 D
10	4×	10.00 D
5	8×	20.00 D
4	10×	25.00 D
2	20×	50.00 D
1	40×	100.00 D

Table 10.2: Magnification and lens power scheme at a reference distance of 25 cm.

Distance of object (in cm)	Magnification	Lens needed
25	1×	4.00 D
12.50	2×	8.00 D
6.25	4×	16.00 D
5	5×	20.00 D
2.50	10×	40.00 D
1	25×	100.00 D

the object is held. This is one of the reasons why working in diopters rather than magnifications when describing aids is more meaningful.

ANGULAR MAGNIFICATION

Angular magnification is the magnification experienced when looked through binoculars or telescopes. It is created by a system of lenses in the telescopes. When the object is too far away or too large to move closer or just too big to change its size, angular magnification is needed. The telescope lenses bend the light ray so that when they leave the telescopes, they appear to be coming from the same direction as an object closer to the eye, thus the object appears much larger.

$$\text{Magnification} = \frac{\text{Angle subtended by image}}{\text{Angle subtended by object}}$$

Figure 10.3 shows that the light rays enter the telescopes and instead of leaving in the same direction they enter and form a normal image, the telescopic lenses increase the convergence of the rays and the rays enter the eye as through coming from an apparent object sitting much closer to the eye than the real object. Thus, the brain perceives the object as being bigger and closer and greater detail is seen.

The telescopes are useful for distance objects that cannot be enlarged or moved closer. However, it has a limited field of view and has motion parallax. Thus, a telescope is used mainly to spot objects rather than full time wear.

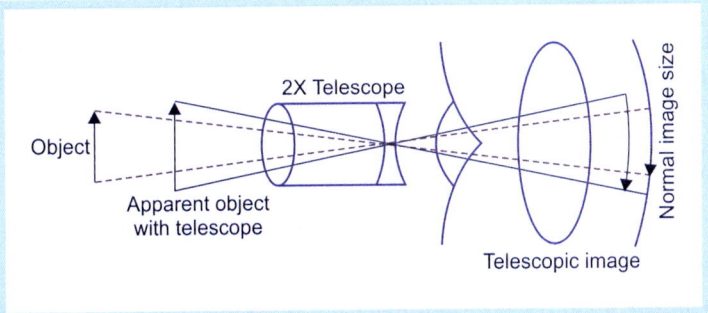

Fig. 10.3: The telescopic lenses increase the convergence of the rays and the rays enter the eye as if coming from an apparent object sitting much closer to the eye than the real object. Thus the brain perceives the object as being bigger and closer and greater detail is seen.

PROJECTION MAGNIFICATION

Under the projection magnification, the enlargement of an object is achieved by projecting it onto a screen, such as in films, slides, and so on. The most familiar aid that utilizes this principle is the closed circuit television system (CCTV). The aid creates magnified image using one or more magnification systems. When two types of magnifications are combined, the total magnification is the product of the two systems.

$$\text{Magnification} = \frac{\text{Size of screen image}}{\text{Size of the image}}$$

POWER OF MAGNIFICATION

The degree to which the viewed object is enlarged is the power of magnification and is usually expressed by a number followed by "X." This symbol is used to express power or the size of the object in relation to its actual size and is derived from the refractive power of the lens.

Historically, it has been assumed that the "distance of most distinct vision" is 25 cm or 10 inches, i.e., if a normal person is interested in seeing an object as clearly as possible with the unaided eyes, he should hold it at a distance of 25 cm. This is being designated as a magnification of 1. The standard presbyopic and emmetropic patient needs a +4.00 D lens, which has a focal length of 25 cm to see an object clearly at the distance of most distinct vision. Therefore, +4.00 D lens is said to have a magnification power of 1× and thus the equation can be derived as:

$m = D/4$

where, m = magnification
D = dioptric value of the lens

This equation holds true only if the object is placed at the primary focal distance of the plus lens.

Example: A simple plus lens gives the magnification for 3×, what is its dioptric value?

$m = D/4$,
$3 = D/4 = 12.00\ D$

PREDICTING MAGNIFICATION REQUIRED

Predicting the magnification required implies that we can select a suitable magnifier more quickly, although the prediction is only a general guide to start the work up for magnification requirement. In each case, the optimum spectacle distance should be in place while the predictions are made. It may not significantly affect the performance and may be discarded later.

Distance Magnification

For a distance task, we must try to estimate what acuity would be required to perform a task adequately. For example, 6/18 acuity may be needed to watch the television or 6/6 to read the bus number.

$$\text{Magnification required} = \frac{\text{Required visual acuity}}{\text{Present visual acuity}}$$

For example, to improve the visual acuity from 6/60 to 6/6 on Snellen chart:

Magnification required = 60/6 = 10×

The same method can be used to assess the improvement which may be achieved with a particular device by the following equation:

Achieved visual acuity = Magnification × Present visual acuity

For example, a patient with a visual acuity of 6/36 using 4× telescope would achieve visual acuity of:

$$\text{Achieved visual acuity} = 4 \times 6/36$$
$$= 6/9$$

Near Magnification

To calculate the magnification requirement for near vision, start by measuring the present acuity for reading at near distance. This varies depending upon the position of the material. By convention the standard 1× magnification is achieved by using a viewing distance of 25 cm—the focal length of the standard +4.00 D. This implies that we must test the near vision at this distance with whatever reading addition is appropriate on top of the full distance correction. The reading addition may be zero in a young adult, but the full +4.00 D addition may be needed in an elderly person. The value of addition does not affect the calculation.

To determine the required "target acuity," the patient should be questioned about what they wish to read at the reading distance. Hence, when the initial appointment is made, the patient can be asked to bring the samples of the visual tasks with which they find difficulty and the size can be measured.

The assignment of an acuity level to a nonreading task, such as knitting or wiring a plug, is even more difficult. It can be estimated and achievement of the acuity is confirmed with the reading chart, but the magnification required should then be "fine-tuned" with the actual requirement.

For near point chart:

$$\text{Magnification required} = \frac{\text{Present visual acuity}}{\text{Required visual acuity}}$$

For example, if the patient could read N 20 at a standard distance of 25 cm and wanted to read N 5 print, then the magnification required:

$$\text{Magnification required} = 20/5$$
$$= 4\times$$

The reading performance with this magnification can be checked using a high plus trial lens in front of the eye. In our above example using +16.00 D lens, the patient should be able to achieve N 5 when reading chart is positioned at the focal point of the lens, i.e., 6.25 cm from the lens.

SELECT THE CORRECT ANSWER

1. A patient uses a 12.00 D lens as a simple magnifying glass. What is the resultant magnification?
    a. 2×
    b. 3×
    c. 4×
    d. 6×

2. Which of the following low vision aids utilize the principle of projection magnification?
    a. Telescope
    b. Hand magnifier
    c. CCTV
    d. Stand magnifier

3. Large print text and felt tip pen are the examples of which of the following magnification principles?
    a. Relative size magnification
    b. Relative distance magnification
    c. Angular size magnification
    d. Projection magnification

4. When an object is too far from the patient, which of the following magnifications works to magnify the object size?
    a. Relative size magnification
    b. Relative distance magnification
    c. Angular size magnification
    d. Projection magnification

Answers

| 1. b | 2. c | 3. a | 4. c |

SELF-PRACTICING QUESTION

1. Illustrate the difference between angular magnification and projection magnification.

11 CHAPTER

Illumination

Chapter Outline
- Sources of Illumination
- Ways to Help Patient with Illumination Control

There are three important factors to the performance of any visual tasks which are shown in **Flowchart 11.1**.

Illumination is very important among all the environmental factors and the importance of illumination system increases while working with visually impaired patients. Illumination can improve the functioning of optical aids or even has potential to replace the need for optical aids. Illumination increases visual function by:
- *Reflection of light from the object*: The human eyes see the object when the light falls on the object, reflected from it, and then transmits to the eye. The simple rule is higher illumination is needed for efficient seeing. If most light is absorbed by the object, it makes the object darker or opaque.
- *Enhancing contrast*: The ease of seeing an object depends a lot on its contrast with background and neighboring objects which depends upon the illumination falling on the object and

Flowchart 11.1: Factors to the performance of a task.

1. The task itself
2. The person performing the visual task
3. The environment which the visual task is performed

its reflection factor. Visual performance varies directly with the contrast level and illumination required varies inversely with it.
- *Reducing glare*: Too much illumination in the peripheral field of view reduces the visual efficiency by creating a veiling effect and thus reducing the acuity.
- *Improving visual comfort*: A balanced illumination is important for comfortable visual performance which means distribution of light is equally important.

The need for illumination in low vision care is patient dependent, depending upon:
- *Age of the patient*: Older population in general requires more light than the younger population. Visual resolving power begins to fall past mid-life. Retinal illuminance of a 20-year guy is three times more than that of 60 years' person. There is a steady loss of visual efficiency after the age of 20 years in terms of speed and acuity in addition to the accommodation power.
- *Ocular condition*: Media opacities and optical irregularities result in light scatter within the eye. Nuclear sclerosis produces yellowing of lens and thus prevents shorter wavelength of light reaching the retina.
- *Visual task*: The intensity of illumination varies inversely with the size of detailing required. The brightness of an object is equal to its illumination multiplied by its reflection factor. It implies that with the same degree of illumination, visual efficiency will be different for different tasks such as reading on white paper, sewing gray cloth, or working on black velvet.

There are lots of advantages that can be availed by illumination control in low vision rehabilitation; some of them are as under:
- Illumination reduces the need for magnification.
- Illumination minimizes glare and maximizes contrast.
- Less tiring for the patient as the patient can maintain natural posture.
- Allows the patient necessary flexibility of easy alteration of illumination level
- Greater sense of accomplishment as the patient works more like a normal person

There are two basic sources of illumination:
1. Natural light
2. Artificial light

Natural day light is considered to be the best from psychological point of view but the application of natural light is reduced in modern days because of indoor working environment where artificial lights need to be installed to provide adequate and uniform light to perform visual task. Artificial lights are of different types.

SOURCES OF ILLUMINATION

Incandescent light

Incandescent lights are more directional and have its main spectral output in longer wavelengths. It generally provides more contrast.

Halogen light

Halogen lights are high-intensity lights and are available in smaller and portable lamp types. In reality, they may present some concern because of its cost, thermal effect, and ultraviolet (UV) output.

Light-emitting Diode

Long-lasting, energy efficient, and inexpensive, light-emitting diode technology has gobbled up half of the general lighting market in a decade. Light-emitting diodes (LEDs) produce more light than incandescent lamps. New research has shown that the "blue light" in LED lighting can damage the eye's retina and disturb natural sleep rhythms.

Neodymium light

Neodymium bulb emits much less UV and blue light than incandescent bulbs. Much of the yellow portion of the visible spectrum created by an incandescent light source is filtered out, leaving illumination with the appearance of blue/white daylight.

Fluorescent Light

Fluorescent lights are mostly used in modern offices and also at home as they are energy efficient and cost-effective. Since the spectral output is in the blue portion of the spectrum, it is often considered harsh. Patients often complain of discomfort glare which can be minimized by using diffusers or indirect installation.

WAYS TO HELP PATIENT WITH ILLUMINATION CONTROL

There are three different ways in which low vision patient can be helped by illumination control:
1. Illumination quantity
2. Illumination quality
3. Illumination distribution

Illumination Quantity

Human eyes can function with considerable degree of efficiency over a large range of illumination. Therefore, in assessing the intensity of light required for a given task, the visual acuity required to do the task should not be made the criterion, instead it can be determined subjectively wherein accuracy, speed, and absence of fatigue can be considered.

Illumination Quality

The two factors that should be considered are flickering of light and color. Flickering lights excites rapid changes in adaptation and is considered as psychological annoyance. The visual efficiency is highest with white light and fatigue has been said to come more readily with red and yellow light than with blue and green light.

Illumination Distribution

The distribution of light is important in two respect—avoidance of glare and to ensure balanced distribution of light. To avoid glare, sources of light should be as far as possible outside the line of vision. Care should be taken to ensure that the eyes do not get the reflected lights also. When surroundings are of markedly different brightness from the working area, there is a great reduction in visual performance. The visual performance increases if surrounding illumination is increased to the level of a little below the test objects. Light from oblique sources increases background illumination—causing glare and poor contrast.

From the functional point of view:
- The position of light source is more important than the actual wattage of light. Light should be adjusted on the object and should not shine in the eyes.
- The light source should be directed over the shoulder of the better seeing eye and held close to the reading material to get maximum illumination.
- The bulb should have an air-cooled shield surrounding it to protect the patient from its heat and to eliminate glare.

Illumination control is very important in low vision management as light increases contrast. Glare is the light that is not useful. It comes from oblique sources and enters the periphery of the eyes, thus increases background illumination and reduces contrast. It is, therefore, important to consider the illumination control devices with the optical aids. A goose neck lamp or flexible arm lamp can be extremely beneficial as it can be positioned such that the illumination is optimal for a given task.

However, not all patients need much light, the need for which depends upon factors as mentioned before. The examiner must consider those factors and prescribe proper illumination. Illumination can be said to be the amount of light falling on the surface or the object. The measuring unit is "lux" when the distance between the light source to the surface is measured in meters. It is "foot candles" when the distance between the light source to the surface is measured in feet. 1 lux is equal to 0.0929 foot candles, whereas 1-foot candle is approximately 1 W.

Chapter 11: Illumination

SELECT THE CORRECT ANSWER

1. Which of the following ocular conditions is not benefitted by minimizing the illumination level?
   a. Albinism
   b. Aniridia
   c. Age-related macular degeneration (ARMD)
   d. Polycoria

2. Which of the following is more relevant illumination control mechanism that can be applied for low vision patient's improved visual performance?
   a. Illumination quality
   b. Illumination quantity
   c. Illumination distribution
   d. All of the above

3. Illumination control for distance vision includes all of the following except.....
   a. Side shields
   b. Typoscopes
   c. Tints and coatings
   d. Multiple pinholes

Answers

| 1. c | 2. c | 3. b |

SELF-PRACTICING QUESTION

1. Write a note on how illumination control works for low vision patients. Give examples.

CHAPTER 12

Low Vision Aids

Chapter Outline

- Optical Aids
- Nonoptical Aids
- Spectacle Lenses as Low Vision Aids
- Visual Field Expanding Aids
- Contact Lens as Low Vision Aids
- Advanced Low Vision Aids
- Computer-Assisted Devices
- Assessment for Computer-Assistive Devices

One of the most common perception is that the magnifiers are the only aids that can be prescribed for low vision patients to improve their visual functioning. To some extent, it is true as most aids that are prescribed use the principles of magnifications in one or other manner. But this is not completely true as a credible job can be performed with great effectivity with many other devices.

For the purpose of simplification, we can categorize different low vision aids that are available in six broad categories as shown in **Flowchart 12.1**.

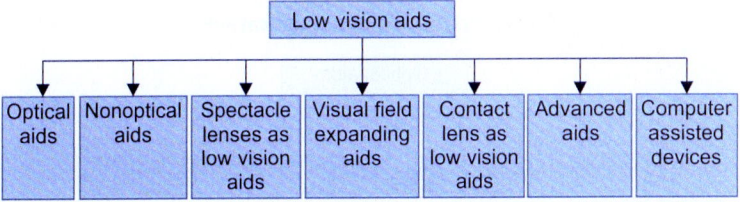

Flowchart 12.1: Different types of low vision aids.

OPTICAL AIDS

Optical aids are considered to be the most imperative tools of the low vision aid practice. Optical aids must be prescribed by the low vision practitioner after thorough low vision examination as only prescriptive optical aid provides desired visual functioning. **Flowchart 12.2** shows the main types of optical aids that are commonly prescribed in low vision aids practice.

Microscopic Lenses

A low vision microscope can be described as a spectacle mounted convex lens. They function on the principle of relative distance magnification. When considering a microscopic lens, the following options may be tried:

Full Field Microscopes

Full field microscopes are mounted in conventional frames and are used at a normal vertex distance. They may be developed in several lens designs such as spherical lens, aspheric lens, and doublets.

Half Eye Microscopes

Half-eye microscopes (**Fig. 12.1**) are convex lens mounted in a half-eye frame worn at a distance little longer than normal vertex distance. The greatest advantage of the half-eye microscope is unobstructed distance viewing. Classic half-eye microscopes are convex spherical lens with base in prism designed for binocularity. The usual amount of prism incorporated into each lens is equal to the power of the plus diopter. For example, a +8.00 D half eye would have 8.00 D of base in prism before each eye.

Flowchart 12.2: Types of optical aids.

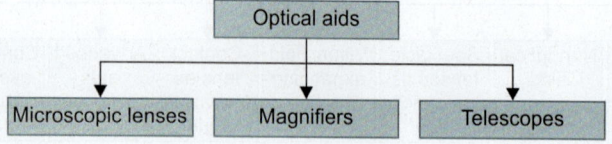

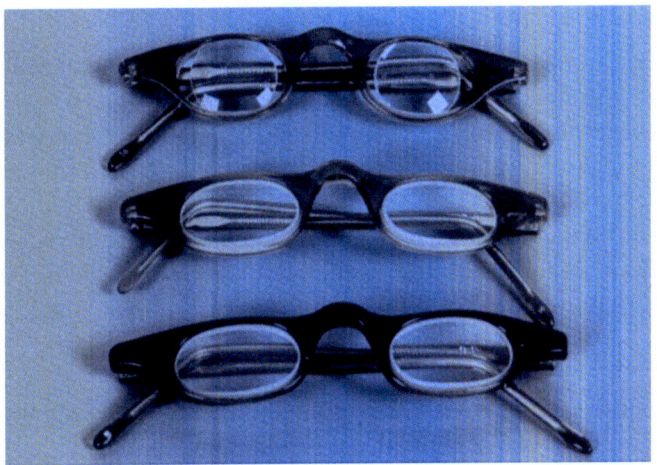

Fig. 12.1: Half-eye microscopic lenses.

Bifocal Microscopes

Bifocal microscopes are mounted in conventional frames and are used at a normal vertex distance. The segment height depends on the patients' needs and the power of the bifocal. Microscope lens allows both hands to remain free and is useful for prolonged reading. It also provides largest field of view. But it decreases the working distance.

Magnifier

Magnifiers are designed to help the low vision patients with the short-term spotting of tasks at near while using the current reading glasses. Magnifiers have been used as vision enhancing device for countless years. The basic principle underlying the use of magnifiers is to provide an increased image size that covers a larger area of the retina. This increased image coverage of the light sensitive retina, compared to the unmagnified image, allows the brain to interpret the image more easily. A magnifier is a primary aid of choice for many patients as it solves most of their reported problem. It may also be an excellent secondary aid, for example, a patient may use a spectacle microscope for reading but rely on a handheld magnifier for checking prices for shopping.

General Principles of Magnifier

- The stronger the power of the lens, the smaller is the diameter.
- The stronger the lens, the closer it must be to the paper.
- The greater the magnifications used, the smaller the area viewed.
- Stronger lens reduces the transmission of light, and thus more light may be required.
- The direction of a magnifier faced may make a big difference.
- The closer the eye is to the magnifier, the wider is the field of view.
- High powered lenses have a lot of peripheral aberrations.

Types of Magnifier

There are several types of magnifiers. **Flowchart 12.3** shows the different types of magnifiers available.

In each category, these magnifiers can range in power from 2× to 10×. Lower powered magnifiers are larger and as the power increases, the width of the lens reduces.

Handheld Magnifier

The handheld magnifiers (**Fig. 12.2**) are the most common visual aid. The object to be viewed should be held at the focal distance of the magnifying lens.

For example, if a 5×, i.e., +20.00 D lens is used, the object should be held at 5 cm (100/20 cm = 5 cm) from the magnifier. At this distance the light rays leave the magnifier at zero vergence. This implies that the individual can hold the magnifier at any distance from the eye and still enjoys the same level of magnifications, no accommodation is needed. The field of view may be larger if the magnifiers are held closer to the eye. Handheld magnifiers can also be illuminated where they serve as an excellent ancillary aid for certain situations where light is difficult to control like in hotels or at nights, etc.

Flowchart 12.3: Types of magnifier.

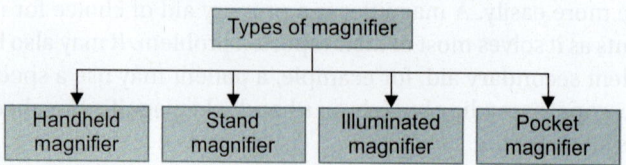

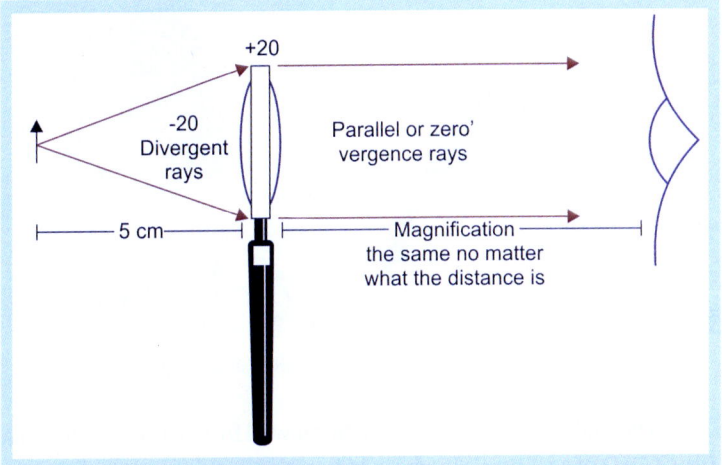

Fig. 12.2: When an object is held at the focal distance of a handheld magnifier, the light rays leave the magnifier at zero vergence.

Features
- Handheld magnifiers are more suitable for short duration tasks, but for longer period of reading, the patient may have difficulty in maintaining the focal length.
- Since closer to eye use of magnifier is desired to increase the field of view, this inevitably makes them monocular unless the lens is very large.
- Handheld magnifiers may be of various shapes and sizes depending upon their power and purpose.

Stand Magnifier (Fig. 12.3A)

Many patients prefer the stand magnifier because it is relatively easier to use. The stand automatically sets the magnifier at the correct distance from the reading material. The stand magnifier may be illuminated or nonilluminated and focusable or nonfocusable. A nonfocusable stand magnifier is a convex lens in a rigid mounting that has been set by the manufacturer closer to the page than its focal distance to reduce peripheral aberrations. Therefore, the rays emerging from the stand magnifier are no longer parallel but divergent, requiring accommodation effort or a moderate reading addition to bring the image into focus.

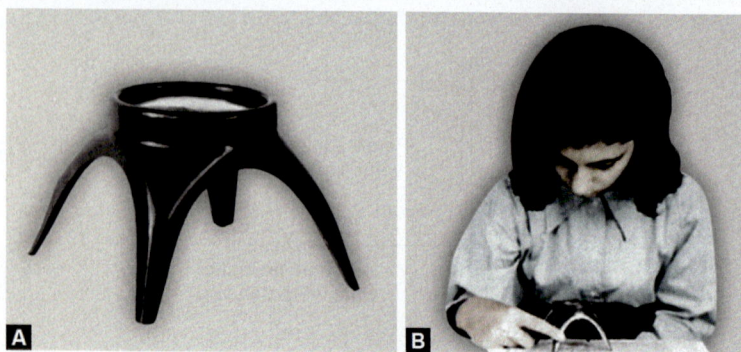

Figs. 12.3A and B: (A) Nonfocusable stand magnifier.

This virtual image is intended to be viewed from a normal distance with +2.50 D of addition. However, in practice patients generally prefer stronger addition to get closer and gain a wider field. The advantages of fixed focus stand magnifier are as follows:
- Predictable focus with rigid lens mounting
- Reading distance relatively normal
- Useful for specific short-term detail tasks
- Useful for children
- May be used with a standard reading addition

The disadvantages of fixed focus stand magnifier are as follows:
- Reduced field of vision
- Posture may be awkward and tiring.
- Less aberrations occur if the image is viewed from an angle.

The focusable units can be used to correct simple refractive errors. It is a good alternative for the patients who cannot tolerate the critical reading distance of strong spectacles or hand magnifiers. The eye is kept very close to the lens of the focusable unit.

The advantages of the focusable stand magnifier are:
- No accommodation is required and is useful for the patients who have rejected magnifiers or spectacles because of difficulty in maintaining focal distance.
- The disadvantage of the focusable stand magnifier is the restriction in the field of vision.

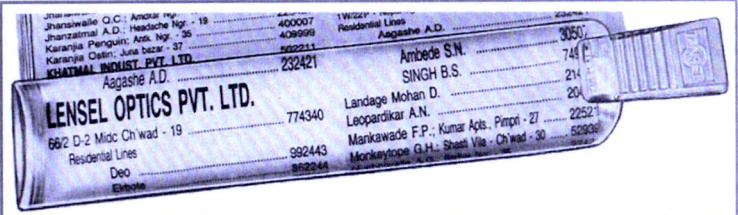

Fig. 12.4: Bar magnifier.

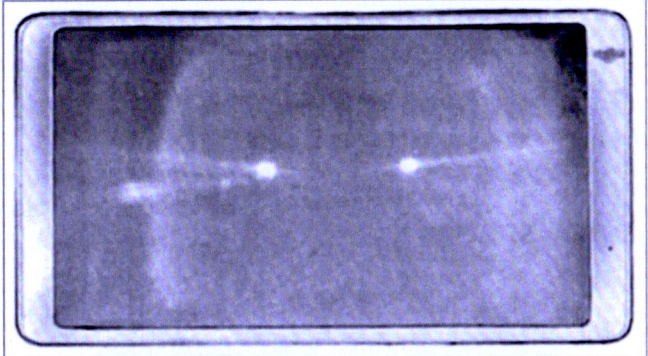

Fig. 12.5: Fresnel magnifier.

Bar Magnifier

A bar magnifier (**Fig. 12.4**) is a cylinder reading bar which lies flat on a page. It elongates the letters but does not separate them. It thus magnifies only in the vertical direction. A person with a small central field who needs minimum magnification may benefit from this optical property. Bar magnifiers are usually available in low magnifications only.

Fresnel Type Magnifier

A Fresnel lens magnifier (**Fig. 12.5**) is in the form of a thin plastic and finds application in subnormal vision practice as handheld magnifier. The lens surface is reproduced in a series of rings or zones which are impressed into the face of the material and by this method of manufacture, spherical, elliptical, and parabolic surfaces may be produced in an inexpensive manner in almost any size. The number of rings per inche controls the resolution and effective magnifications which may be as high as 10× for ophthalmic purposes. The principal advantage of Fresnel lens is that they are extremely light weight. But the definition and quality of the magnified image is rarely as good or bright and field correction is also not extensive.

Telescopes

Telescopes (**Fig. 12.6**) are the only aids that improve the resolution of a distant object by enlarging the image using angular magnification. In their simplest construction, a telescope contains two optical elements—objective lens and eye piece. In all the telescopes designed to provide angular magnification, the objective lens is positive in power and is placed toward the object to be viewed. The eye piece, placed close to the eye of the observer, is much stronger in power than the objective lens and may be either a positive or negative lens.

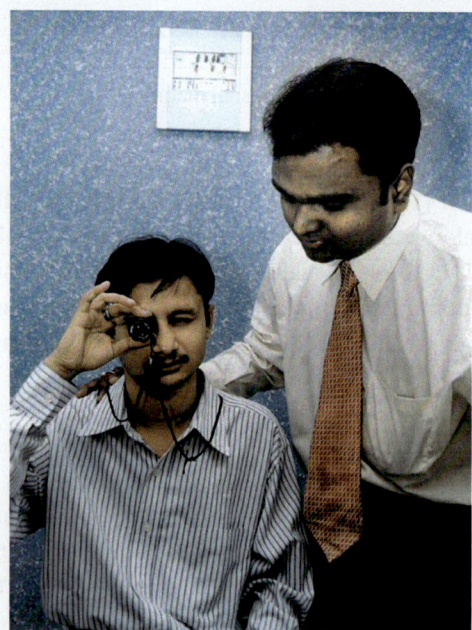

Fig. 12.6: Telescope.

There are two types of telescopic systems for low vision patients as shown in **Flowchart 12.4**.

Galilean Telescope

A Galilean telescope, also known as Dutch telescope, is a simple system of a convex objective lens combined with a concave ocular lens that produces a real, upright image when the lenses are separated by the difference in their focal lengths. The concave ocular lens always has the higher power. Rays that leave the systems are parallel when the secondary focal point of the objective lens coincides with the primary focal point of the ocular lens. The size and location of the exit pupil determine the light transmission and field of view of the telescope. In Galilean telescope, the exit pupil is usually located inside the telescope. Galilean telescope used for low vision may be focusable or nonfocusable.

The magnification of Galilean telescope is determined by the ratio of ocular lens power to the objective lens power and is given by the following formula:

$$\text{Mag (GT)} = -\frac{D_{(Ocu)}}{D_{(Obj)}}$$

Example: If the lens power of the objective lens of a Galilean telescope is +16.00 D and the lens power of the ocular lens is –36.00 D, find the magnification produced by the telescope.

$$\text{Mag (GT)} = -\frac{-36}{16}$$

$$\text{Mag (GT)} = 2.25 \times$$

The length of the tube of the Galilean telescope is determined by the algebraic summation of the focal length of the objective lens and the focal length of the ocular lens and is given by the following formula:

Flowchart 12.4: Telescopes.

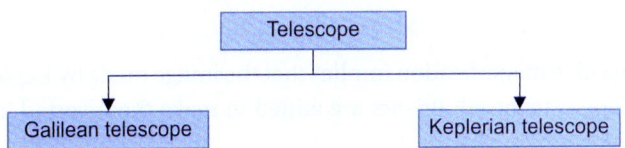

d = F(Obj) + F(Ocu)
Where d = Tube length
F(Obj) = Focal length of the objective lens power
F(Ocu) = Focal length of the ocular lens power

Example: If the lens power of the objective lens of a Galilean telescope is +16.00 D and the lens power of the ocular lens is –36.00 D, find the length of the tube.

$$d = (100/16) + (100/-36)$$
$$d = (6.25) + (-2.78)$$
$$d = 3.47 \text{ cm is the tube length}$$

Keplerian Telescope

In a Keplerian telescope, also known as prismatic telescope, both the objective lens and ocular lens are convex lens. An internal system of a prism erects the inverted image. The image quality and brightness across the field of view are usually better in Keplerian telescope than Galilean telescope. The field of view through a Keplerian telescope is usually large and they are available in higher magnifications than Galilean design.

The magnification of Keplerian telescope is determined by the ratio of ocular lens power to the objective lens power and is given by the following formula:

$$\text{Mag (KT)} = -\frac{D_{(Ocu)}}{D_{(Obj)}}$$

Example: If the lens power of the objective lens of a Keplerian telescope is +16.00 D and the lens power of the ocular lens is +36.00 D, find the magnification produced by the telescope.

$$\text{Mag (KT)} = -\frac{36}{16}$$

$$\text{Mag (KT)} = -2.25\times$$

Negative magnification implies that the image made by Keplerian telescope is inverted. Prisms are added to make the inverted image upright.

The length of the tube of the Keplerian telescope is determined by the algebraic summation of the focal length of the objective lens and the focal length of the ocular lens and is given by the following formula:

d = F(Obj) + F(Ocu)
Where d = Tube length
F(Obj) = Focal length of the objective lens power
F(Ocu) = Focal length of the ocular lens power

Example: If the lens power of the objective lens of a Keplerian telescope is +16.00 D and the lens power of the ocular lens is +36.00 D, find the length of the tube.

d = (100/16) + (100/36)
d = (6.25) + (2.78)
d = 9.03 cm is the tube length

Full Field Telescope

The full field telescopes cover the entire lens in the frame. Although it gives a larger field of view than the bioptic telescope, it is used only for visual activities that may be accomplished while standing or sitting because learning to walk with this type of the lens is difficult and should only be attempted in the presence of an experienced low vision instructor.

Telemicroscopes

Telescopes are focused for distance objects. They cannot be used for near objects as they do not allow accommodation. However, some telescopes are designed so that its ocular lens can be moved outward, creating the effect of plus power to focus on near objects. A telemicroscope is simply a telescope with reading cap incorporated into its frontal, i.e., objective lens **(Fig. 12.7)**. The power of the reading cap dictates the working distance. Since the goal is to have zero vergence rays entering the telescopes, the material must be placed at the focal point of the reading cap. The magnification changes with the different reading caps. For example, with a 4.00 D cap, the magnification of the telemicroscope is equivalent to the power of the telescope. Reading cap stronger than +4.00 D will increase

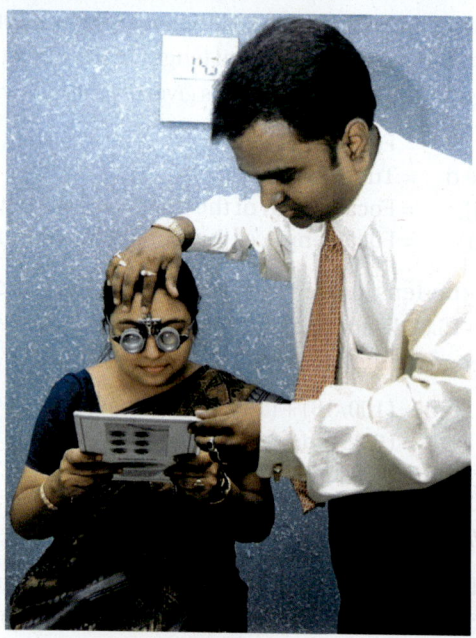

Fig. 12.7: Telemicroscope.

the magnification and power less than +4.00 D will decrease the magnification. The magnification can be determined by the following formula:

(Power of telescope) × (Diopter of cap/4) = Power of telemicroscope

Telemicroscopic lens provides greater working distance than microscopic lenses but they sacrifice the field of view.

Bioptic Telescope

When a person needs a telescope for constant use and yet is always moving about, a bioptic telescope (**Fig. 12.8**) may be prescribed. This type of telescope uses conventional plastic ophthalmic lenses in a frame and a small hole is drilled in the top part of the lens and a miniature telescope is mounted in each hole. The conventional lens is used for general viewing and the bioptic telescope is used for seeing distant object in details. To use the bioptic telescopes, the person

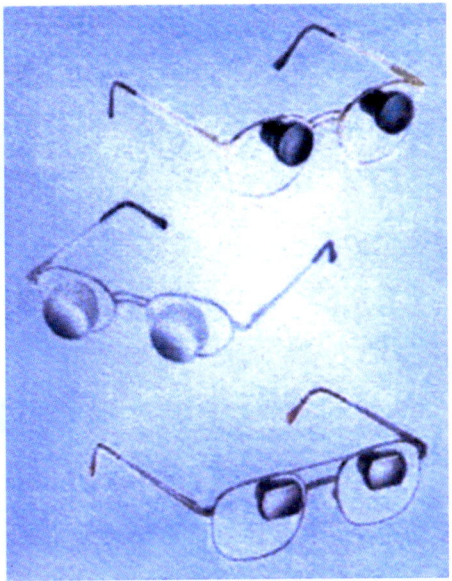

Fig. 12.8: Bioptic telescope.

lowers the head and raises the eye to look through the telescope portion. When he does not need the telescope, he raises his head and continues, looking through the conventional lenses.

NONOPTICAL AIDS

Nonoptical devices play an important role in the successful use of many optical low vision devices. They complement, supplement, or substitute for optical aids. Often nonoptical devices are used alone also. They work by altering the environmental condition of the low vision patient. They are of following types which are described below.

Large Print

Large print **(Fig. 12.9)** involves the concept of using relative size magnification. If an object is made larger, it will be easier to see.

The amount of magnification obtained depends on a comparison of the new larger object compared with the standard size object. The advantages of using larger print lie in its easy acceptance by the low

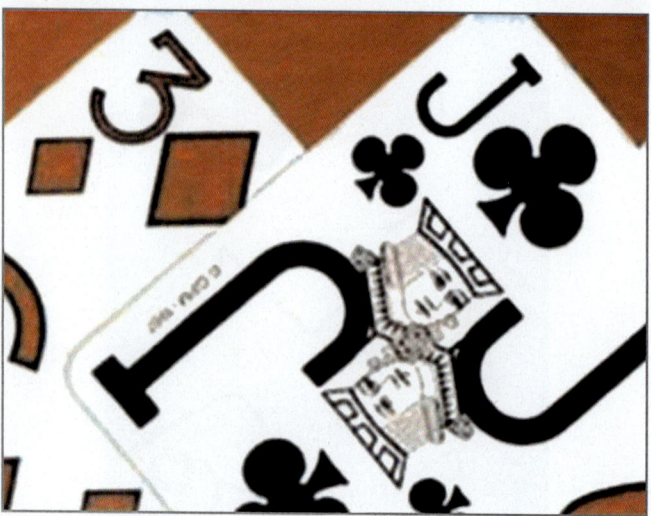

Fig. 12.9: Large letter cards.

vision patient. Large print is sometimes used along with low power optical device to provide the proper combined magnification. One major disadvantage of large print is that of limited magnification. It is common for large print books not to exceed 18 points, which provides 1.8× magnification only. With this amount of magnification only a small segment of the low vision population can rely solely on large print alone.

Illumination

Proper illumination **(Fig. 12.10)** is essential for the low vision patient. Light should be adjusted on the printed material and should not shine in the eyes. Illumination can be thought of as light that strikes the material to be viewed and bounces back directly into the eye. This light increases contrast or increases the difference between the light coming from the object viewed and the light level of the background of the object. Glare is the light that is not useful, it comes from oblique sources and enters the periphery of the eye, thus increasing the background illumination and decreasing contrast. As glare decreases contrast and causes fatigue and strain, it is important to consider

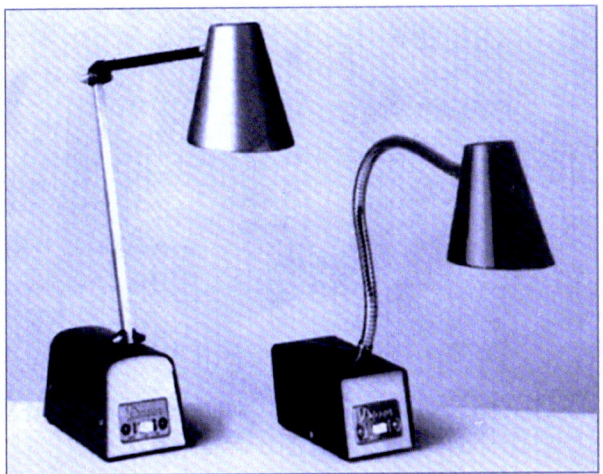

Fig. 12.10: Table lamps.

illumination control devices with all optical aid systems. A goose-neck lamp or a flexible arm lamp can be of tremendous benefit. However, all patients do not need much light. Therefore, the low vision specialist must decide as to the most comfortable level of light for the patient.

Black Felt Tip Pen

The black felt tip pen instead of blue ball point pen can be used to enhance contrast which is necessary for reading printed materials. With felt tip pen, one can also write larger to give a magnified image.

Typoscopes

A typoscope **(Fig. 12.11)** is a piece of black card board with a slit in it. It blocks out all but the line of print viewed through the slit. When a single line print is framed by a black, that line tends to stand out better and appear sharper, thus increasing the contrast.

Reading Stand

The purpose of a reading stand **(Fig. 12.12)** is to hold the reading material in a comfortable position so that the patient can maintain a close working distance without straining the neck and back muscles or

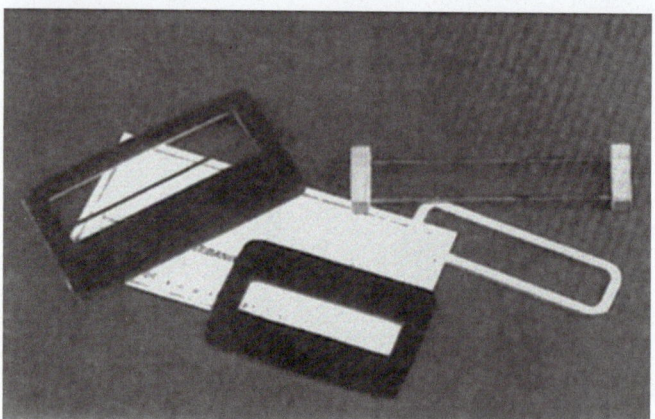

Fig. 12.11: Typoscope.

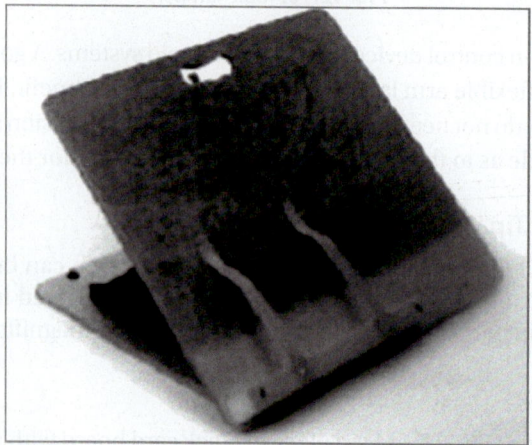

Fig. 12.12: Reading stand.

tiring the arms. Many people add one adjustable lamp to help reading, especially for extended periods. The reading stands may also be used to reduce the object distance to ensure magnification effect.

Visors and Caps

Visors and caps can be used to provide protection from the sunlight.

Talking Products

Talking books, talking watches, talking calculators, talking telephones **(Fig. 12.13)**, etc., are a few of common devices that are available with speech output. Often many of these voice-output products also have large display incorporating relative size magnification along with voice output. This combination makes for an extremely useful product.

Tactile Products (Fig. 12.14)

The second largest sensory input that is used when the visual sensory input is not functional is the sense of touch. Braille is the most common type of product to provide this sensory input.

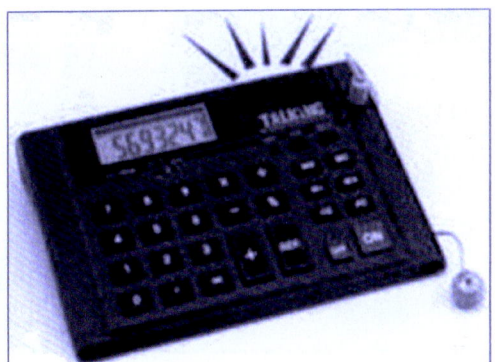

Fig. 12.13: Talking telephone.

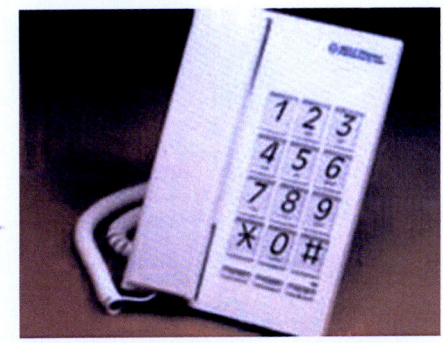

Fig. 12.14: Tactile telephone.

Needle Threader

Needle threader (**Fig. 12.15**) is also a nonoptical aid to carry out a specific task like threading a needle.

Notex

Notex (**Fig. 12.16**) can be designed to help identifying the different notes.

Night Vision Aid

Nightscope or simply a torch light may be used for additional illumination in the night while movement.

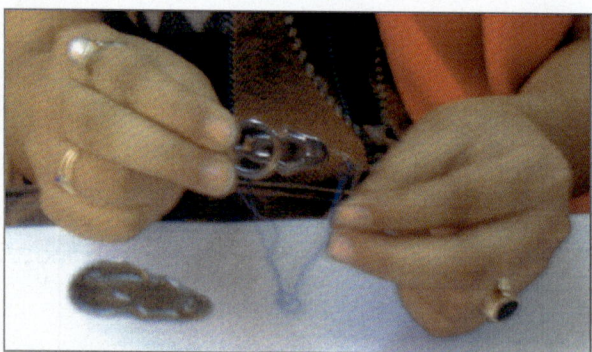

Fig. 12.15: Needle threader.

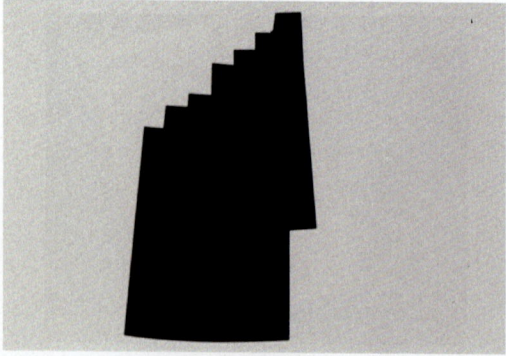

Fig. 12.16: Notex.

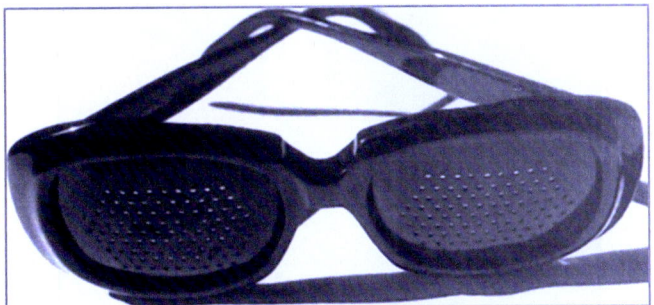

Fig. 12.17: Pinhole spectacle.

Pinhole Spectacle

Single or multiple pinhole (**Fig. 12.17**) spectacles are sometimes useful for lens opacities, pronounced vitreous opacities, and for corneal scars. Pinhole spectacles are not made of glass at all but of an opaque substance such as metal or plastic. The user looks through any of the small holes in the material. These holes have the effect of reducing the width of the bundle of diverging rays coming from each point on the viewing object. Thus, they cut out peripheral beams and glare and any refraction error in the lens or cornea is not noticed as much. It is better to control the size of aperture by trial and error method. When any sort of reduced apertures is prescribed, the amount of illumination lost must be compensated. It must also be remembered that increased illumination causes greater pupil contraction.

SPECTACLE LENSES AS LOW VISION AIDS

Absorptive Lenses

Poor visual acuity is not the only problem with low vision. Glare and contrast enhancement present new and different challenges for the low vision clinicians. Low vision absorptive lens (**Fig. 12.18**) should have properties to absorb ultraviolet (UV) light. Some absorptive lenses, which are actually filter, can make a scene appear to be darker or brighter, screen out specific colors, or provide increased contrast without altering colors. Colored lenses have their greatest effect on opposite colors, for example, a red lens transmits red light but absorbs or blocks blue and green light. The use of red filter by a low

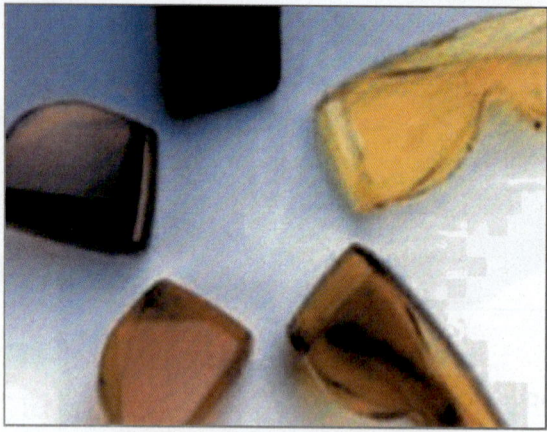

Fig. 12.18: Absorptive lenses.

vision patient may cut out blues and green. A green lens blocks red or orange light; a yellow filter blocks blue light. An orange or yellow filter used on a gray day may give the impression of sunshine. Neutral density lenses reduce the amount of light reaching the eye without altering the color. These lenses may be desirable for patients whose chief complaint is photophobia or intolerance to light. Patient who complains of red-deficient fluorescent light may respond favorably to yellow, orange, or red filters. All yellow, orange, and red lenses in general increase contrast for patients whose major problem is mobility in poor contrast. For low vision patients, the potential benefits of absorptive lenses are removal of discomfort glare, reductions of veiling glare, improved adaptation to changes in illumination, and improved contrast and/or acuity. Various types of absorptive lenses are available for the low vision patient in glasses as well as plastics. They are as described below.

Noir Filter

Noir medical technologies manufacture an extensive line of plastic filters of several transmissions in both goggles and frames styles. The Noir UV shield styles offer a variety of transmission with complete UV blockage while the Noir filter styles offer complete UV as well as significant infrared reduction.

Corning Photo Chromatic Filters

The development of corning photo chromatic filter (CPF) lenses is an attempt to design a filter to provide protection of eyes in cases of progressive retinal degenerations.

Younger Protective Lens Series

The younger protective lens series have also developed filter lens that would protect the eyes by filtering UV and short-wavelength blue light.

Antireflection Coating

An anti-reflection coating is applied to the lenses to prevent the reflection of light and enhance light transmission to the eyes. It helps the user see and feel better compared to uncoated lenses. Many low-vision patients require a very steep or very flat curvature. These lenses may produce reflections that may affect the clarity and resolution of the vision as a result. Anti-reflection coating also minimises the effect of internal reflection, which may be more pronounced, especially when the lenses are thick. Back surface reflection, which occurs when the lights hit the back surface of the lens from behind and reflect back into the eyes, is also very annoying for the eyes. An anti-reflection coating is subtly applied to the lens surface. The film blocks reflections coming in from the front and back. Tinted lenses are used as absorptive lenses in low vision practise to reduce glare and improve contrast. The darker the tint, the more glare is blocked out. Applying the anti-reflective coating on the back surface of tinted lenses may be more helpful to block out glare and unwanted reflection. In fact, anti-glare and anti-reflective lenses work slightly differently, but they both have the same aim: to block out unwanted and annoying light.

VISUAL FIELD EXPANDING AIDS

Field expansion aids offer a variety of options for individual with reduced visual fields. There are three options available to an individual who wishes to compensate for a larger area of missing field as shown in **Flowchart 12.5**.

Flowchart 12.5: Three types of field expansion devices.

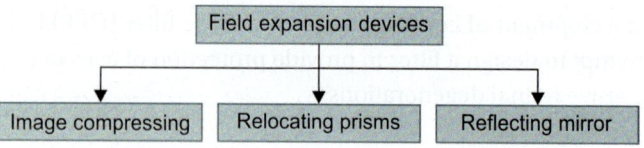

Relocating Prisms

Relocating prisms are very useful in the management of patient with visual field loss. The base of the prism is placed in the direction of nonseeing area of the eye which causes the image shift toward the apex which lies in the direction of retina where there is residual vision. For example, in patient with hemianopic temporal field loss, the base of the prism is placed toward the temporal area and apex toward the nasal area. When the patient glances into the prism, he does not have to look far toward the blind side because the image has been displaced nasally onto the seeing retina. Thus, the patient is able to reduce the eye movement. The amount of prism is determined by clinical trial and the amount of prism is decided based upon patient's goals, amount of peripheral field loss, and adaptation to the displaced image.

Fresnel Prism

Fresnel prisms (**Fig. 12.19**) are pliable soft plastic lenses that can be temporarily attached to a regular spectacle lens. Fresnel prisms can be placed over the entire lens or just out from the midline into the area of field loss. When the individual directs his eyes into the prism area, lower contrast image from the missing field will come into view. Because of the decrease in visual acuity as a result of the reduced contrast, most individuals will reject Fresnel prisms as a permanent solution for field enhancement. However, a trial is helpful to see if the individual would benefit from having a prism incorporated into a spectacle correction. The commonly used prism diopters are 15 D, 20 D, and 30 D.

Field-expanding Channel Lens

Field-expanding channel lens is useful for patients with retinitis pigmentosa and glaucoma. Inwave optics has developed a lens

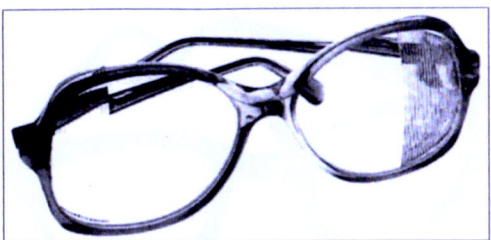

Fig. 12.19: A Fresnel prism placed base out in each spectacle lens.

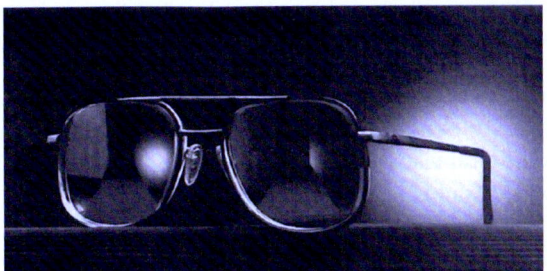

Fig. 12.20: The inwave field-expanding channel lens.

system that has two lateral prisms on either sides and one prism at the inferior portion of the lens with apex of each prism lying toward a central nonprismatic channel (**Fig. 12.20**). The prescription can be incorporated into the front surface of the lens and the lens system can be designed for various degrees of peripheral field loss.

Image Compressing

Image compressing is the process of minifying the image size and compressing them within the useful field of vision. This is a kind of field enhancement for sighting. The concept of sighting means the patient observes while in stationary position. The gadgets which are commonly used as image compressing tools are described below.

Reverse Galilean Telescope

Reverse Galilean telescope has been used to enhance the effective visual field for the patients who have peripheral field loss. With this technique, the individual looks through the objective lens of the telescope rather than the ocular lens. Reversing the telescope allows

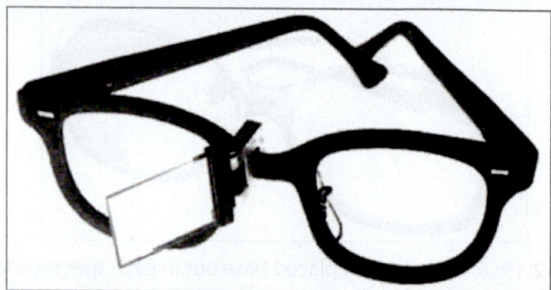

Fig. 12.21: The semi reflective planomirror placed on the nasal aspect of the spectacle frame would aid a patient with a right temporal field loss.

the user to view an entire setting because the image is not magnified, but minified. To benefit from its use, however, the individual must have good central visual acuity and reduced peripheral fields, as is the case with patients who have retinitis pigmentosa.

Handheld Concave Lens

Handheld concave lens can also be used as sighting device for patients with constricted visual field.

Reflecting Mirror

Monocular hemianopic mirrors (**Fig. 12.21**) have been used to reflect an image from a nonseeing area into the seeing field of view.

CONTACT LENS AS LOW VISION AIDS

Contact lenses for low vision patients have considerable applications in both young and old patients. Provided it is rightly exploited, they can offer distinct advantages over other low vision aids, and in many cases, they are more effective. Both corneal and haptic contact lenses are employed in subnormal vision practice.

Contact Lens for High Myopes

Patients who have progressive or pathological myopia can often obtain good clinical results when fitted with contact lenses. A spectacle lens may not provide acceptable quality of vision because of aberrations, distortions, problems with image sizes, or other optical phenomenon.

Contact Lens for Albinism

Glare and photophobia are common complaints encountered in albino patients. These patients frequently display a pendular nystagmoid movements of their eyes as they attempt to use their maculas. This type of movement may also reduce vision. The pinhole contact lens **(Fig. 12.22)** made with an opaque periphery and clear pupil can be used to control rays of light without unduly restricting the field of vision. The nystagmoid movement is also slowed down which may improve the visual functioning.

Contact Lens for Aniridia

Special prosthetic lenses are available for these situations to reduce the photosensitivity problem occurring in patients with aniridia.

Contact Lens for Keratoconus

Keratoconus is a noninflammatory protrusion or ectasia of the cornea in which it becomes thin and distorted. It is usually bilateral, with one eye progressing ahead of the other. The cornea becomes so irregular that quality of vision cannot be improved with spectacle lenses. Contact lens provides immediate advantage because it acts as a "new" cornea or refracting surface.

Contact Lens for Loss of Color Vision (Fig. 12.23)

Occasionally a contact lens can be used to enhance color perception. The patient having difficulty with red and green may be fitted with a special type of lens called X-Chrome lens. X-Chrome is a red contact

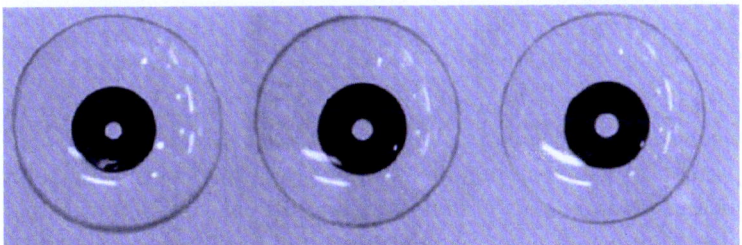

Fig. 12.22: Pinhole contact lens.

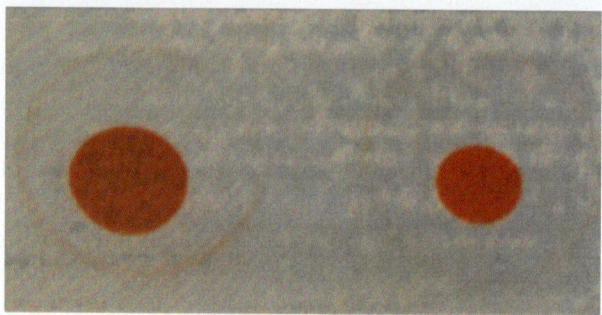

Fig. 12.23: X-chrome contact lenses.

lens that is worn on nondominant eye, though this is not always the case. Its principle is to create what is referred to as retinal rivalry, which enables brain to distinguish between various shades of color.

Contact Lens as Telescopic System

A contact lens may be used to design a Galilean telescopic system. The high-powered concave contact lens works as the eyepiece or ocular lens of the telescope and the spectacle of lower-powered convex lens is worn over it which is used as objective lens of the telescope. The total magnification of the system can be determined by the ratio of the dioptric power of the contact lens to the dioptric power of the spectacle lens.

ADVANCED LOW VISION AIDS

Revolutionary innovations have brought several distinctly new and advanced low vision aids. Some of the popular among them are described below.

Closed-Circuit Television

Closed-circuit television (CCTV) **(Fig. 12.24)** is an example of electronic magnification system for reading used by visually impaired patients. A CCTV system incorporates the principle of projection magnification. A CCTV permits the low vision patient to visually assess printed or handwritten material and a multiplicity of the objects by means of a magnified image projected onto a monitor screen.

Chapter 12: Low Vision Aids

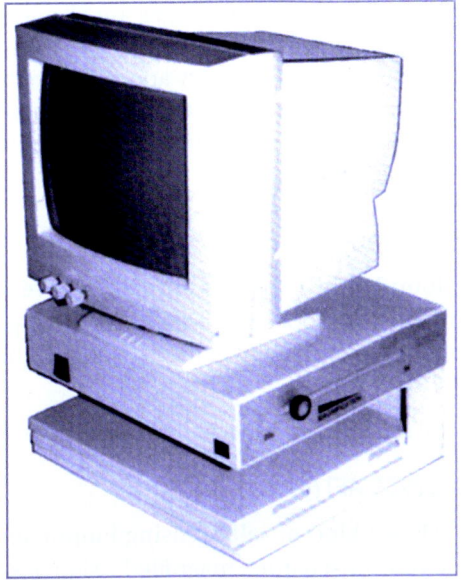

Fig. 12.24: Closed-circuit television.

The standard CCTV consists of three major components—camera, monitor, and movable reading platform. The video camera is directed at an object and the image of this object is projected on a television monitor screen. The monitor serves as the screen onto which the enlarged print image is projected. The movable platform sits on a flat table or a desk and the material to be read is placed on the platform, which is designed to be positioned underneath the camera. All CCTVs enable the patient to select regular polarity, i.e., black letters on a white background or reverse polarity, i.e., white letters on black background for reading. In addition to the polarity change, some black and white CCTV systems have a "photo mode"—when selected, reverts the camera to present contrast and brightness mode that is ideal for viewing photos. The CCTV magnification level ranges from 4× to 65× with some variations in the screen size system. The advantages of CCTV system are as follows:
- Brightness and contrast controls are available.
- Photographs may be easily viewed.
- Binocularity is possible even with larger amounts of magnification.

However, the following disadvantages are also associated with the CCTV:
- Physical size may hinder portability and maneuverability.
- Training and practice time is needed to become a proficient user.
- Limited availability of maintenance services for components
- Initial cost is very high.

Ocutech Vision Enhancing Systems

Ocutech, Inc, founded in 1984, has developed several innovative high quality bioptic telescopes for visually impaired patients. They are used by thousands of visually impaired patients throughout the world **(Fig. 12.25)**.

There are several models available which are described below.

VES®-Autofocus (VES-AF) (4×)

Ocutech VES-AF is a kind of self-focusing bioptic telescope. The VES-AF provides the most natural magnified vision possible because wherever you look, the image will be clear right away, just like natural vision. It removes the most inconvenient parts of using a bioptic telescope-focusing, and the most fatiguing-having to hold still to keep the image in focus. The VES-AF includes a 4× Keplerian telescope that is coupled to an eye-safe computerized infrared autofocusing

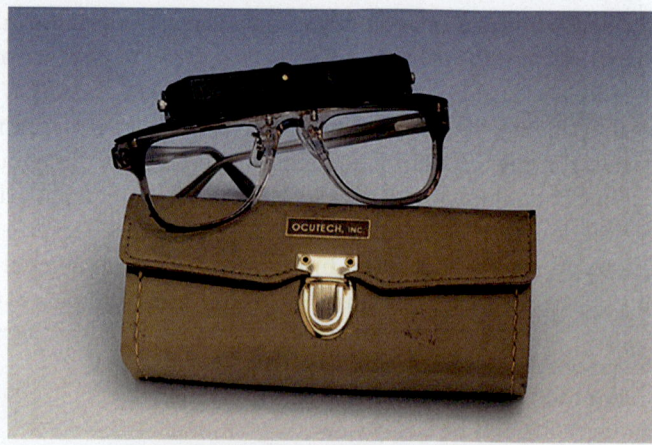

Fig. 12.25: Ocutech bioptic telescope.

system. It measures the focusing distance over 30 times per second to provide a clear image immediately and at any distance as close as 12 inches. This naturally clear vision allows the visually impaired to work much more efficiently and in a much more relaxed and comfortable posture. A rechargeable battery pack operates the VES-AF all day long.

Ocutech VES® II (3×, 4×, 6×)

The Ocutech Vision Enhancing System (VES-II) is based upon Ocutech's original innovative bioptic telescope system, developed and tested with funding from the National Eye Institute. Its design successfully addresses the major drawbacks of conventional bioptic telescope systems, field of view, appearance, weight, and positioning control, which undermine their acceptance by patients and pose fitting problems to prescribers. The VES-II bioptics offer a wide field of view, a bright image, light weight, and easy focusing. The fully adjustable mounting design makes prescribing a high quality bioptic system quick, convenient, and readjustable at any time. Even challenging eccentric viewing and nystagmus patients are now easy to fit.

Ocutech VES® Mini (3×, 15°)

This is one of the smallest, lightest, widest field bioptic telescope. The Ocutech VES-Mini is an innovative, miniature 3× expanded field (Keplerian) bioptic telescope system. It provides a combination of an unusually wide 15° field-of-view in a very compact physical design. The Mini's crisp, bright optics provide internal focusing for refractive errors from +12 to −12 and for near viewing to as close as 7 inches. The convenient diagnostic kit makes it easy to demonstrate and prescribe this high quality telescope system with a minimum of time, effort, and risk. The VES-Mini is prescribed as any other conventional bioptic telescope system and can be ordered for monocular or binocular use and for distance and near applications. It can be ordered mounted in Ocutech's fashionable ophthalmic frames as a complete package, or it can be installed into appropriate frames provided by the prescriber.

Ocutech VES®-K (3×, 4×, 6×)

The VES-K manual focus bioptic telescope offers Ocutech's quality Keplerian optics, that provide a sharp edge-to-edge image and the widest field-of-view available, in a small, light, and comfortable physical design. Patients can wear the VES-K all day long. The VES-K innovative bridge mounting design provides full control of critical telescope positioning, making it easy to demonstrate, fit, and dispense. Even challenging eccentric viewing and nystagmus patients can be fitted with ease. And, the VES-K is easy to readjust or to change carrier lenses at any time.

COMPUTER-ASSISTED DEVICES

The development of computer-assisted devices for low vision patients has the potential to remove many of the limitations of the traditional low vision aids. With specialized assistive equipment, patients with low vision can use the home computer to convert digitized text into a format that compensates for any degree of visual impairment, enlarging text on a screen or converting it to speech. With the computers, the patient can locate specific information using search or find functions and type his message and correspondence. Once the information is found, the patient can gather the information by listening them. Financial and banking transactions can be conducted with computers. Newspaper and magazines are available on the Internet or on commercial on-line information services. Thus, the personal computers have become important assistive devices that allow for accessing and processing information. Four types of adaptation may enable them to use a computer as low vision device as shown in the **Flowchart 12.6**.

Flowchart 12.6: Computer-assisted devices.

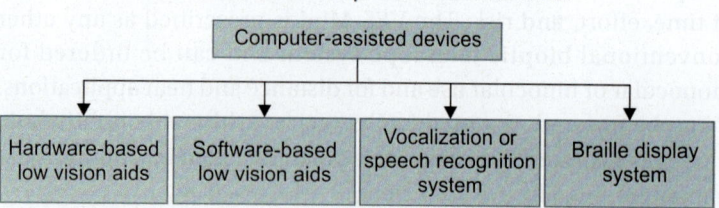

Hardware-Based Low Vision Aids

Large print keyboard **(Figs. 12.26A and B)** has been designed for individuals who suffer from macular degeneration, visual impairments, or just have a hard time reading the commands on the keyboard. The keyboard is offered in several layouts with either multicolored or white keys. Besides, touch screen **(Fig. 12.27)** devices are placed on the computer monitor or built into it that allows direct selection or alteration of the computer by touching the screen itself. The quality of the monitor can greatly affect the clarity of text. The higher resolution monitor screen can be derived for various patients with visual impairment. The display size of the monitor screen can be enlarged to use greater magnifications more effectively. For example, when a subject switch from 14-inch monitor to 21-inch monitor, he is able to achieve an increase in magnification of 1.5×. Patients with certain visual impairments are sensitive to glare on the monitor. For them antiglare treatment can be provided to alleviate

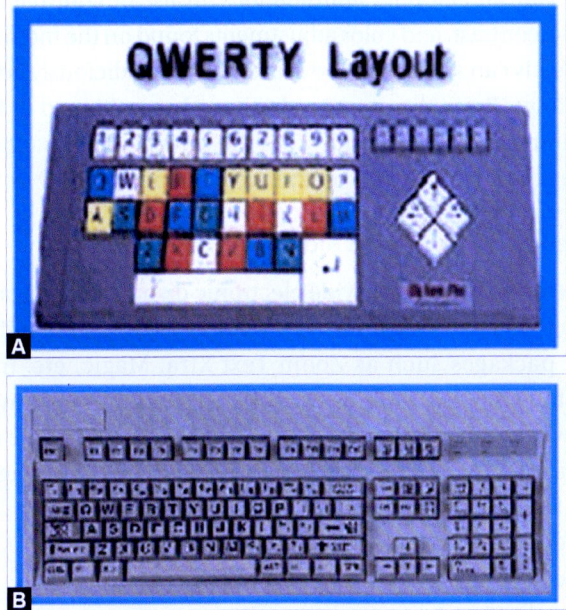

Figs. 12.26A and B: A. Multicolored or white keys; B. Large print keyboard

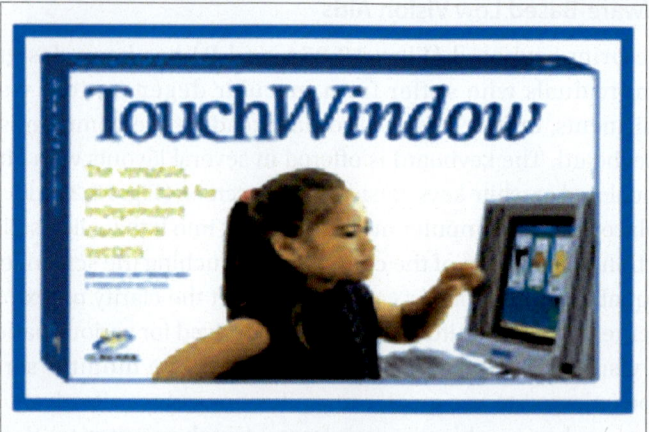

Fig. 12.27: Touch screen.

some of their problems. For those patients who find that antiglare treatment reduces the brightness of the display, separate filters can be used. Glare and monitor illumination can also be controlled by the brightness, contrast, and color adjustments found on the monitor. The patient needs can sometimes be met simply by judiciously adjusting these settings. Fresnel type prism lens can be positioned in front of the monitor at a given distance from the screen which is capable of increasing the character size on the screen approximately by 2×.

Software-Based Low Vision Aids

Many operating systems provide electronic display magnification by increasing the character font size. Special electronic magnification software packages such as Zoom Text Xtra, Magic, etc. magnify text and the graphics. Various other kinds of software are available that allow more tracking and color changes also. Electronic display magnifications through the use of software has many advantages over the use of optical devices. It can:

- Provide greater range of magnification
- Provide contrast enhancements
- Provide luminance control
- Provide reverse contrast

- Modify font types and letter spacing
- Change the color combination of characters
- Permit a greater working distance

Vocalization or Speech Recognition System

It is not necessary to absorb all information visually. In fact, speech system should not be considered as a last resort or only for those with severe vision loss. It can be considered for patients with moderate vision loss also because some patients can read as quickly and comfortably with a speech system as a normally sighted computer user can read visually, whereas other patients prefer visual reading to listening even if they are slower in the overall task. Choice of speech is very much a matter of individual preference. There are two components to all computer speech system—a speech synthesizer and a screen reader. The speech synthesizer translates digital text to speech, much like a printer translates digital text to print. A speech synthesizer requires a piece of hardware that plugs into the computer and a speaker that plugs into the speech synthesizer. A screen reader is a software program that enables the patients to select which portion of the text, displayed on the screen, will be read by the speech synthesizer. An example of using a speech synthesizer and screen reader can be seen with a patient who wishes to enter a certain command into his word processing program. As the patient types the command, the screen reader relays each letter typed to the synthesizer, which in turn speaks each letter as it is typed. The patient also has the option of typing the entire word, sentence, or paragraph and then striking a key combination to instruct the synthesizer to read the entered command aloud. The patient is also able to speed up the reading rate or change the voice from male to female using commands to the screen reader. In addition, the patient has the ability to ask the screen reader to pause and spell a word that is not recognized or to have it phonetically pronounced. The primary problem associated with vocalization systems is their inability to access graphics and patients' difficulty in navigating an application. Still the patients with some functional vision may benefit from combining electronic magnification with vocalization systems.

Braille Display Systems

Braille is the tactile substitution for gathering information (**Fig. 12.28**). The system of reading and printing consists of raised dots that are tactually identified. The pattern of dots represents letters or symbols that have been almost universally accepted by the blind individuals. Some patients with severe visual impairment may choose braille for correspondence because it empowers them with information processing ability that is both quick and accurate. Given letters or the combination of letters is represented by a specific configuration of dots. In fact, it is a kind of shorthand system. Braille can be typed into a computer by the use of a braille keyboard. This special keyboard uses only six keys, and each key corresponds to one dot of the braille cell. Thus, by pressing some combination of keys, any letter or letter combination can be created. Braille system has the capability of translating standard word processing material directly into braille format. In addition, for individual who are not familiar with braille, written print can be typed into a computer and is automatically converted to braille and read by a visually impaired patient on a braille output device or is embossed onto braille paper. Braille printers require software that translates the printed signal to the appropriate braille character. A braille output device is a braille display system with "refreshable"

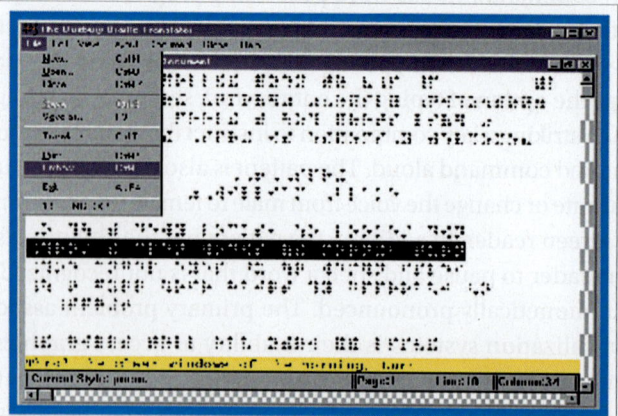

Fig. 12.28: Braille translation software.

braille cells. With a refreshable braille device, a series of braille characters is electromechanically "flattened." Once the individual has read the information, the next set of braille cells automatically pop up as the braille output device continues to translate the printed material on the computer.

ASSESSMENT FOR COMPUTER-ASSISTIVE DEVICES

Evaluating a patient for a computer-assistive device may be considered a three-step process:
1. A low vision assessment
2. A computer specialist's assessment
3. Instructions

During the low vision assessment, the practitioner in conjunction with the patient establishes the need for the computer-assistive device. Once it is established, the low vision practitioner should determine the need for optical magnification, electronic display magnification, a speech system or possibly some combination thereof. If an optical device is involved, the practitioner should determine the appropriate amount of magnification along with the type of device and working distance.

In the computer assessment, the computer specialist should demonstrate and help to configure the complete computer system by recommending specific components that are compatible with one another as well as being compatible with the patient's needs. The recommended computer components should also be based on the low vision practitioner's recommendations and any optical devices that the patient expects to use with the computer system. The final process in this triad technical assessment program is instruction. The patient should be provided with adequate instruction in the assistive components that are required for efficient use of the computer system as well as instruction in the software application program. This service can be provided by various professionals such as rehabilitation teachers, or computer specialists.

Some of the popular software for visual impaired patients are described below.

MAGic Magnification Software

MAGic Magnification Software enlarges the image on the monitor screen from 2 times to 16 times its normal size that enables the low vision patients to use the computers. It is available in two types:
1. MAGic without speech
2. MAGic with speech

Jaws (Fig. 12.29)

"Job Access with Speech" is a blind user-friendly talking software that converts a normal computer into a talking computer so that the visually impaired who have lost vision to a large extent or have only light perception where only magnification cannot help, can operate the computer independently.

Big Shot Screen Magnifier (Fig. 12.30)

Big shot screen magnifier magnifies the screen while a low vision patient is working. 20 steps of magnifications from 105 to 200% with changing magnification facility using mouse is possible.

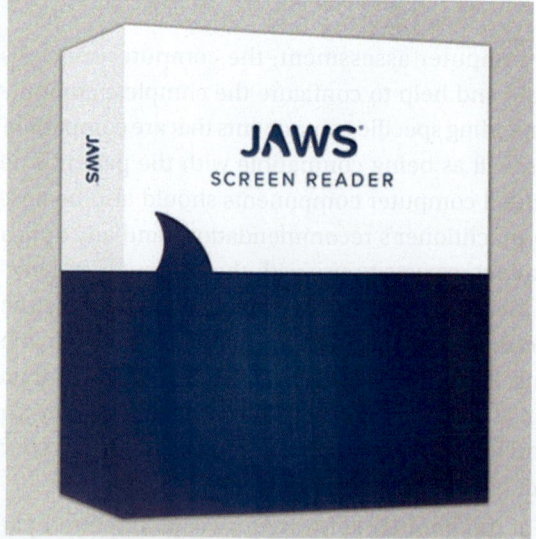

Fig. 12.29: Jaws screen reader.

Chapter 12: Low Vision Aids

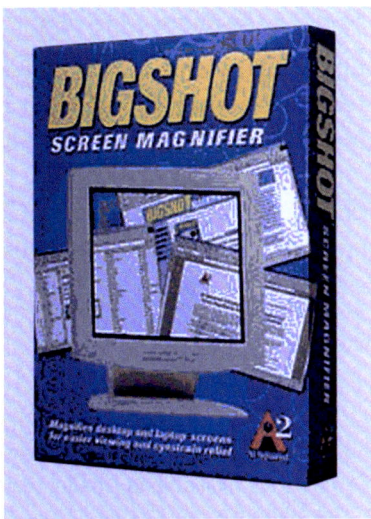

Fig. 12.30: Big shot screen magnifier.

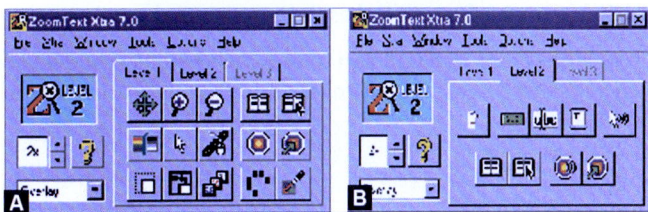

Figs. 12.31A and B: A. Level 1 toolbar; B. Level 2 toolbar.

Zoom Text Xtra (Figs.12.31A and B)

This is the most advanced screen magnifier available in the market today. It is available in two types:
1. Zoom text Xtra level 1
2. Zoom text Xtra level 2.

Level 1 provides magnification from 2× to 16× with color filtering for improved contrast and readability. Level 2 features synchronized magnification with screen reading that is powerful and easy to use. It also speaks all on the screen text, echoes typing, and automatically reads multipage document.

Mobile Speak Talking Mobile Phone Software

This converts a regular mobile phone into a talking one, thus enabling the visually impaired to have complete access to all features of the phone that allow the user to use mobile phones independently.

SELECT THE CORRECT ANSWERS

1. Which of the following is not considered under the category of optical aids?
   a. Spherical half eye lenses
   b. Hand magnifier
   c. CCTV
   d. Telescopes

2. Which of the following is not true about hand magnifiers?
   a. Stronger magnifiers are available in smaller diameter
   b. The stronger the magnifier, the farther it must be to the paper
   c. The most curved side (Cx side) of the magnifier lens is held toward the patient's eyes
   d. Greater magnification makes the areas viewed smaller

3. An objective lens of a Galilean telescope is +30.00 D and its ocular lens is –75.00 D, which of the following suggest the tube lens of the telescope?
   a. 2.00 cm
   b. 2.20 cm
   c. 3.00 cm
   d. 3.33 cm

4. Which of the following suggests the dioptric power of the ocular lens of a telescope when its tube length is 3.00 cm and the objective lens power is +25.00 D?
   a. +50.00 D
   b. –50.00 D
   c. +25.00 D
   d. –25.00 D

5. Which of the following is not the common reason for prescribing absorptive lenses to a low vision patient?
   a. Removal of glare
   b. Improved contrast
   c. Improved adaptation to changes in illumination
   d. For protection from UV rays

Chapter 12: Low Vision Aids

6. Which of the following is not true about Fresnel prism?
   a. It results in poor contrast
   b. It is free from distortion and aberration
   c. It causes reduction in acuity
   d. It is attached to spectacle lenses by surface tension only

7. CCTV is based on the principle of...
   a. Relative size magnification
   b. Relative distance magnification
   c. Angular magnification
   d. Projection magnification

Answers

1. c	2. b	3. a	4. b	5. d
6. b	7. d			

SELF-PRACTICING QUESTIONS

1. Write a short note on Braille Software System.
2. Write a short note on the application of prism in the management of low vision patients.

CHAPTER 13

Prescribing Low Vision Aids

Chapter Outline
- Prescribing Near Viewing Aids
- Prescribing Distance Viewing Aids
- Prescribing Aids for Visual Field Defects

Once all the tests have been done and predicted reading addition is determined, the examiner needs to evaluate to see whether the results work for the patient to meet his visual objectives. This is done by demonstrating the appropriate low vision aids. Low vision aids are available in many forms. While prescribing the low vision aid, the practitioner must consider the following three set of factors in his mind:

Patient and the Patient's Visual Goals

A low vision patient uses an aid only when it serves his visual needs and continues using them when they are easier and simple to use and also hassle free and handle. Therefore, the practitioner must keep following factors in his mind:

- That the established visual habits will tend to dominate in spite of visual impairment which means if the patient is customary wearing spectacle, he will tend to accept stronger reading glasses for his low vision aids. Patients who have already adapted to pocket magnifier or hand magnifier may easily adapt to stronger magnification.
- Unlike routine eyeglass prescriptions, most low vision devices are task-specific. As a result, many patients with low vision are prescribed more than one device for their daily tasks. Ninety percent of patients require reading aids. However, some

younger patients may also need distance viewing aids. The understanding is that patient's visual goals as set during history taking should be kept in mind.
- Finally, the practitioner should also keep in mind patient's general health, financial conditions, and his preferences.

Test Results and the Visual Aids

The low vision practitioner must consider following factors while prescribing low vision aids:
- The results of the tests of visual function.
- The amount of magnification required for the target print size or object size, as determined during the low vision examination.
- The optical properties of the device being considered.

Practice Objectives

The main challenge in low vision practice is not just to prescribe the visual aid once only but also to keep provisions for changing future needs. A good practitioner, therefore, also sets up his practice objectives which he always tries to achieve while prescribing low vision aids, these are:
- The visual condition of the patient may worsen with time. It means that the practitioner must rely more on simple aids than on complex and more expensive aids which may be preserved for future needs.
- A decrease in the magnification prescribed either by using illumination or by adding nonoptical aids.
- Patient's mobility, the low vision aid should be light in weight and portable.

Based on patient's visual goals and above factors, the practitioner may start with either reading aids or distance vision aids. Although many types of aids are available, magnifications are primarily used to meet patient's visual objectives.

PRESCRIBING NEAR VIEWING AIDS

All near magnification aids can be grouped into three different categories as shown in **Flowchart 13.1**.

Flowchart 13.1: Different types of aids for near vision.

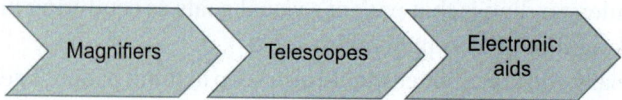

The examiner may use test cards or newsprints or reading material of patient's choice to demonstrate the effectivity of the aid. The patient is instructed to hold the reading material at a very close distance. The examiner starts with magnifiers. There are different types of magnifiers that are often prescribed for reading. They are:
- Spectacle magnifier
- Hand magnifier
- Stand magnifier

Spectacle magnifiers, also known as microscopic lenses, are presented first. They are the most familiar type and accepted form of aids for prolonged reading because of relatively large field and freedom of both hands. Spectacle magnifiers are available as:
- Reading convex sphere in either full diameter or in half eye, also known as microscopic lenses
- Reading convex sphere with base in prism in half eye, also known as microscopic lenses
- Aspheric sphere in full diameter
- Aspheric lenticular lenses
- Monocular clip on loupes

If the patient is not comfortable with full diameter microscopic lenses, he may be asked to try half-eye microscopic lenses. The greatest advantage of half-eye microscopic lens is the unobstructed distance vision. However, with higher power patient finds it difficult to maintain binocularity when he reads at a distance closer than 8 cm. Classic half-eye microscopic lenses with base-in prism are designed for binocularity. The usual amount of prism incorporated in each lens is equal to the power of the plus lenses.

The next aid to explore with the patient is hand magnifier. Hand magnifier can be effectively used with patient's distance correction. However, it can also be used in conjunction with bifocal lenses. In such cases, the need for effective power of the magnifier is reduced. The examiner should not stop when he sees that the patient is responding well with the hand magnifier. He may show unexpectedly improved performance with stand magnifier. Two types of stand magnifiers are available—fixed focus and variable focus. Select a stand magnifier with appropriate power range and support the reading material on a clipboard or a reading stand. Show the patient the correct distance for the specific stand and also how to move the device along the page. Illuminated stand magnifiers are also available that may be used when there is need to increase the contrast level or the patient needs more illumination to read. Focusable stand magnifiers are used for patients who require higher reading addition particularly when spectacle and hand magnifiers are not acceptable. Reading telescopes are demonstrated when a patient requires larger working distance or have some specific vocational requirements such as reading music, typing, or writing. There are different types of reading telescopic lenses are available. Patients usually take time to truly appreciate the usefulness of telescopes. Closed-circuit television (CCTV) is normally considered at last. It is a versatile aid. It provides greater working distance and is demonstrated using familiar reading materials.

Observations

As the patient tries to read using different low vision aids, the examiner must observe and make records for the patient's reaction. Reading is an extremely complex visual task, which involves the integration of visual, cognitive, and motor processes. It is important that the examiner remembers that the reading speed is not very critical to observe in low vision care as long as the patient is able to achieve his visual goals. Four different observations as shown in **Flowchart 13.2** are critical before coming to a decision to prescribe a low vision aid.

Flowchart 13.2: Critical observations by the low vision examiner while demonstrating aids.

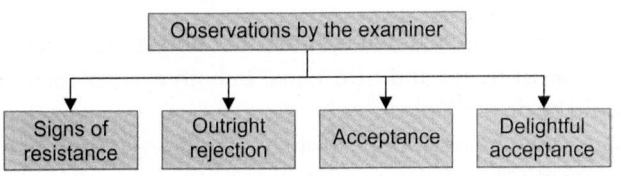

Table 13.1: Factors to observe during reading aid trial.

Difficulties in reading may suggest a need for more magnification
Feeling of dizziness with high plus full field spectacle lens may prompt the idea of trying half-eye spectacle
Difficulties in locating the beginning of each line of the text may suggest the need for typoscopes
Exaggerated hand motion and head turns while using hand magnifier may suggest rejection to hand magnifier
Improvement in reading performance with increase in illumination may suggest reduction in magnification
Lifting of stand magnifiers while trying to read through the same may suggest either the stand magnifier is weak or a hand magnifier is preferred
Reading telescopes are good for extended working distance or for some specific vocational requirements
Bifocal segment in high plus power may interfere with the lower field of vision when the patient walks. This is very critical with constricted field disorders such as retinitis pigmentosa and glaucoma
CCTV should not be the first choice of aid. It should be considered only when all other optical aids have been tried.

(CCTV: closed-circuit television)

Table 13.1 shows some critical factors that should be noted and linked to examiner's observation during reading aid trial.

In case the examiner is not able to relate his observations with patient's reactions, it is prudent to solicit whether or not the patient is happy with the reading performance, provided by the magnifier.

Monocular or Binocular Aid

Most prescriptions for low vision aids are monocular. However, it is a critical criterion before prescribing the low vision aids whether to prescribe monocular aid or binocular aid. There are multiple theories that prevail:
- Some practitioners are of opinion that unless the visual acuity is 20/200 or better and near equal in both eyes, binocular aids should be prescribed.
- There are some practitioners who prefer to prescribe monocular low vision aids in the eye with better contrast sensitivity.

- Some prefer to go by the results of Amsler grid test. The eye with better Amsler grid results is used for monocular aids.

If the visual acuities are similar, then it is always visually beneficial to use the binocular viewing devices. The patient may also feel a psychological benefit from binocular viewing. Unfortunately, the design of the magnifying device or the limitation on the viewing conditions which it imposes may mean that the viewing must be monocular, even if both eyes are open. The reason for this must be fully explained to the patient, who must be assured that ignoring one eye will not cause it to deteriorate, nor will using the fellow eye exclusively cause it to be put under excessive strain. The best approach is to evaluate whether the patient does better monocularly or binocularly. Some patients may perform better when occluding the poorer seeing eye, while other may find it difficult to track the target with monocular aid. In all such cases, binocular aid may be prescribed as they are easier to use than monocular aid to stabilize against the brow, leaving the index finger free to turn the center of the knob.

PRESCRIBING DISTANCE VIEWING AIDS

The philosophy for prescribing low vision aids for distance visual function is totally different. As far as aids for distance viewing are concerned, there are three important criteria which are as follows:
1. Static visual acuity
2. Dynamic visual acuity
3. Photophobia and reduced vision in light

Static visual acuity is more of a concern when the patient is looking at the static target, for example, blackboards in the classroom, sign boards, etc. Dynamic visual acuity becomes more important when the target of concern is at motion, for example, watching sports, following an object, or recognizing the face of a person. Some patients may have reduced visual acuity because of either light scatter inside the eye or because of excessive or unevenly distributed light in the visual environment causing photophobia. While prescribing low vision aids for static visual acuity, magnification becomes more important to the patient, whereas while prescribing low vision aids for dynamic visual acuity, visual field becomes as important as visual acuity. So a balance between the two is desired, the final choice for which is based upon patient's own preference.

There are broadly four types of low vision aids used most commonly as distance low vision aids:
1. Spectacles and contact lenses
2. Absorptive lenses
3. Telescopes
4. Pinhole spectacles

Spectacles by itself do not work for low vision patients. However, they can be effectively used together with contact lenses to provide telescopic effect. Similarly, normal contact lenses are not very effective for low vision patients. But albinism and aniridia patients work very effectively with pinhole contact lenses. X-chrome contact lenses are useful for color deficient patients. Specialty rigid gas permeable (RGP) contact lenses are very useful for keratoconus patients. High minus contact lenses with low plus spectacle lenses can be used to provide telescopic effect.

Absorptive tinted lenses serve double fold purpose as they can protect the eyes and can also enhance the patient's comfort and overall visual performance. Responses to tints are subjective and they must be assessed in different environment both outdoor and indoor before prescribing. It is not appropriate to prescribe the tint on the basis of ocular pathology alone. Traditional tints such as brown, amber, and gray work for low vision care. The enhancement of visual performance through absorptive lenses is because of the reduction in noise that is produced because of light scatter among the shorter wavelengths of light.

Telescope is the only instrument that improves the resolution of distant object by enlarging the image size. There are two types of telescopes used for low vision—Galilean and Keplerian. **Table 13.2** shows the difference between the two types:

There are two main criterions while prescribing telescopes for distance visual function:
1. Field of view
2. Retinal illuminance

Table 13.2: Difference between Galilean and Keplerian telescope.

Galilean telescope	Keplerian telescope
Simple system of convex objective lens combined with concave ocular lens	Both objective and ocular lens are convex. An internal prism erects the image
It provides smaller field of view	It provides larger field of view
It provides relatively poorer image quality	It provides relatively better image quality
They are lighter and shorter	They are heavier and longer
Galilean telescopes are focusable or nonfocusable	Most Keplerian telescopes are focusable
Exit pupil is inside system	Exit pupil is outside system

It is always desirable to have as large field of view as possible while looking through the telescopes. The field of view of telescope is determined by a "field cone" whose angle is determined by the lens aperture size and its distance from the eye.

- The diameter of the objective lenses, larger diameter is associated with larger field of view.
- The size of the exit pupil of the telescope, if the exit pupil of the telescope is larger than the patient's pupil, there is no advantage of prescribing a telescope with larger diameter objective lens. Patients with smaller pupil or glaucoma patients on miotic drops, telescopes with smaller exit pupil would be better. A larger exit pupil in many cases allows the patient to view the object with more ease and better results.
- If the small exit pupil of the telescope is positioned eccentrically in reference to patient's pupil, the field of view through the telescope may appear to be smaller.
- The vertex distance, the field of view is widest when the telescope is held as close to the eye as possible.
- The magnification of the system
- The separation of the objective lens and eyepiece.

Retinal illuminance, or in other words image brightness, commonly understood as light gathering ability of the telescope is another important factor to consider while prescribing telescopes.

Table 13.3: Exit pupil size and retinal illuminance of telescope.

Size of exit pupil	Retinal illuminance
Smaller than eye pupil	Image brightness is reduced
Larger than eye pupil	Image brightness is same as unaided eye
Same as eye pupil	Image brightness is same as unaided eye

Low vision patients are mostly less sensitive to light and need additional lights to achieve a functional vision. The patient's pupil and exit pupil of the telescope play an important role in determining how much light reaches to retina using a telescope. When the exit pupil of the telescope is smaller than the eye pupil, there is reduction in brightness as compared to unaided eye. **Table 13.3** shows the relationship between exit pupil size to light gathering ability of the telescope.

Telescopes can be prescribed as handheld device or they can be spectacle mounted. When a telescope is used for distance spotting task, handheld telescope is commonly prescribed. Longer duration distance tasks indicate a need for spectacle mounted telescope. Handheld telescopes are usually monocular. Some are also available with clips so that they will enable the telescope to be hung on patient's spectacle. The only consideration is they should be available to the patient when they need it. The decision whether to prescribe handheld telescope or spectacle-mounted distance telescope is based upon patient's visual goals, skill, and visual field. Handheld telescopes tend to be preferred as mobility aid whereas spectacle-mounted telescopes are mostly prescribed for school, sedentary viewing such as television watching, etc. A full diameter telescope may be prescribed for sedentary task during which the patient will be looking through the telescope more or less constantly. For tasks involving mobility or intermittent spotting, a bioptic telescopic spectacle (BTS) could be preferred. BTS is composed of two optical elements:
1. A lens with conventional distance prescription
2. A telescope mounted in the carrier lens above the line of sight.

The patient spends most of his time processing information acquired through his conventional lenses and when distance detail information is required, he simply tilts his head or chin down slightly to align the telescope in the straight ahead position.

Patients with aniridia, corneal pathologies, or media opacities are also benefitted by the use of pinhole spectacles under high illumination. These pinholes block indirect rays of light from entering the eye, thus preventing them from distorting your vision. Pinhole, when used in contact lenses, acts as an artificial aperture and improve vision.

PRESCRIBING AIDS FOR VISUAL FIELD DEFECTS

The patient with visual defects mostly reports following symptoms:
- Patients report running into the objects
- Tripping and falling
- Difficulties in detecting objects
- Difficulties in orientation and movements
- Loss of place while reading
- Glare and photophobia

The goal of managing for visual field defects is multifaceted. All treatment and management plan are aimed to improve the patient's overall visual functioning. To achieve the above objectives, following low vision devices are used:
- Fresnel prisms
- Mirrors
- Field expansion channel lens
- Reverse telescope

Central visual field defect or central scotoma is one of the most common visual field defects seen in low vision patients. The scotoma may vary from 1 to 30°. Visual acuity is related to the extent of the disease and the ability of the patient to shift fixation to relatively undamaged parafoveal areas. When a young patient develops macular disease, they usually do not complain of black spot seen in the central visual field, instead they complain that they see better when they look slightly off-center. They learn to view eccentrically almost as a matter of normal process. However, an older patient who develops macular disease continues to use foveal fixation until they realize they see better looking away from the center. They are then taught to look eccentrically or are provided with prism lenses to deflect the image to the healthy retina. Eccentric viewing technique refers to using a nonfoveal location to avoid the central scotoma to obtain the best possible functional vision. The patient may respond well to other devices such as large print materials, increase in illumination, and increase in magnification.

Peripheral visual field defects have more serious functional consequences than central visual field defects. Their total field of vision is constricted that interferes with their mobility more than with reading. The peripheral retina perceives gross objects and movements in the visual periphery, alerts the macula to identify the stimulus, and at night adapts to the dim light vision. They complain that they walk hesitatingly in unfamiliar place and often extend an arm for sensing any obstacle outside their seeing area. They may also report difficulty seeing larger and magnified objects without constant scanning. The use of magnification does not have the desired effect. Reverse Galilean telescope provides more information to these patients by compressing more information into the residual visual field. Inwave Optics, Inc. has developed field-expanding channel lens to improve the mobility with the patient viewing objects through the channel while having the advantage of temporal, nasal, and inferior awareness for retinitis pigmentosa and glaucoma patients.

Homonymous hemianopia is characterized by loss of two halves on the corresponding area of the visual field in both eyes, i.e., either the left or the right half of the visual field. Right hemianopic patients may be prescribed a mirror attached to the nasal eye wire which is angled before the right eye. The mirror blocks out most of the left visual field of the right eye, replacing it with a view of the right visual field. Hence, the left eye in this case views the left visual field, and the right eye views the right visual field through the mirror. Images seen in the mirror are reversed and move rapidly when the head is moved. The patient must learn to suppress the mirror image. It only allows the patient to be aware of what is happening in the right visual field. The patient must make gross eye and head movement to actually look at an object of interest in the blind field.

Bitemporal hemianopsia is the condition of partial blindness where vision is missing in the outer half of both the right and left visual field. These patients have been shown to work well with prisms placed base out at the temporal portion of the lens.

A prism system has been accepted for peripheral field enhancement more than any other system. The benefits of prisms are same as that of mirror. They cause a displacement of an object in the patient's blind area to an area on retina where there is useful vision. A major advantage of prism over mirror is that the prism is placed on the area of eye that is nonseeing and therefore, does not cause an additional blind spot or dual image. The patient is also able to reduce his eye movements. The only fact that the patient must keep in his mind is that the purpose of prism is not to sharpen the image but to enhance the awareness of the peripheral objects.

There are nonoptical aids also that are prescribed either as complementary or supplementary or substitute for optical aids. It is possible that for a particular patient, reading may not be important at all. He may be frustrated more because he is unable to play cards or sign cheques or dial numbers in telephone. Some optical aids may have been introduced during the examination and demonstration process. Some patients may prefer these simple devices more than magnifications.

In addition, for students' low vision patients, the examiner should not forget to make following recommendations:

- Reading aloud when the teacher writes on the blackboard
- Experiment with colored chalk and other media. Green boards are poor.
- No large amount of homework should be assigned. Assign various types of homework instead of great amounts of the same.
- Experiment with contrast and backgrounds. Some children work better on black surface, some on white.
- Tapes are very helpful teaching devices.
- Expect some standard of work, but perhaps, not as much quantity.
- Classroom displays should be at eye level of students.
- Develop positive attitude in both visually handicapped students and teachers. The teacher's attitude is probably the single most important factor in the student's confidence in him.

- Use of good quality nonglare whiteboards, felt tip markers are useful.
- Enlarging print is not always the answer for visually handicapped students. It is limiting. Try magnification by using normal print close to the eyes. Sometimes if a child has a blurred image and you enlarge it, he only sees a bigger blurred image—it does not make it clearer.
- Oral work is important, use spoken language.
- Students should take part in all activities unless restricted by medical doctor.
- Watch for changes in visual behavior.
- Provide concrete materials—models, real items.
- More stress on self-activity and independence on high priority

The examiner must consider these factors before completing the consultation and when the consultation comes to the end, it is important that the examiner does not forget to open the document where he wrote the goals as set at the beginning and should read out to the patient. He must explain what is being achieved and what is not achieved together with justifying reasons.

SELECT THE CORRECT ANSWER

1. Which of the following low vision aids provide greatest working distance for reading?
   a. Microscopic lenses
   b. Magnifier
   c. CCTV
   d. Telescopic lenses

2. While trying microscopic lenses for reading, if the patient finds it difficult to locate the beginning of each line of the text, the examiner may adopt the following course of action?
   a. Patient should be told that the microscopic lenses will not work for you.
   b. Typoscope may be tried together with microscopic lenses.
   c. Microscopic lenses should be kept aside and telescope should be tried.
   d. Any of the above

3. Which of the following is the best approach to take a decision on monocular or binocular reading aid?
   a. If the visual acuity is 20/200 or better and near equal in both eyes, binocular aid should be prescribed.
   b. Monocular aid should be given in the eye with better contrast sensitivity.
   c. The eye with better Amsler grid results should be given monocular aid.
   d. The best approach is to evaluate whether the patient does better monocularly or binocularly.

4. Which of the following is not the features of Galilean telescope?
   a. Provides smaller field of view
   b. An internal prism erects the image
   c. Lighter and shorter
   d. Provides relatively poor image quality

5. Which of the following is not the factor to consider to determine the field of view of a telescope?
   a. The vertex distance of the telescope
   b. The size of exit pupil
   c. The size of objective lens
   d. None of the above

Answers

| 1. c | 2. b | 3. d | 4. b | 5. d |

SELF-PRACTICING QUESTIONS

1. Glare and photophobia are common complaints of most low vision patients. Explain with reasons and recommended management strategy.
2. When demonstrating the reading low vision aids to a patient, how would you decide whether to prescribe monocular low vision aid or binocular aid?

CHAPTER 14

Patient's Training

Chapter Outline

- Training for Distance Viewing Aids
- Training for Near Viewing Aids

Low vision care is much more than a prescription of low vision aid. Training is one of the most integral parts of low vision care. The purpose of training is to help the visually impaired person to use his residual vision more effectively either with aid or without aid to gain functional independence for day-to-day life activities. Effective training helps patient change his self-image from an "impaired person" to a "person with impairment."

Training for the low vision patient has to be approached methodically in a given order that follows the sequential steps as given in the **Flowchart 14.1**.

Near vision training should start with all activities with simple visual tasks and as the training progresses, it should progress into more detailed and confusing visual tasks. The most successful distance viewing training program ideally starts with static objectives while the patient is in sitting, then the patient works with moving objects and the patient works with moving objects and finally, the patient works with moving objects while he is also mobile.

TRAINING FOR DISTANCE VIEWING AIDS

Training for distance viewing technique follows a sequential process that follows the steps in sequential order as shown in **Flowchart 14.2**.

Flowchart 14.1: Step-by-step process for providing training to low vision patient.

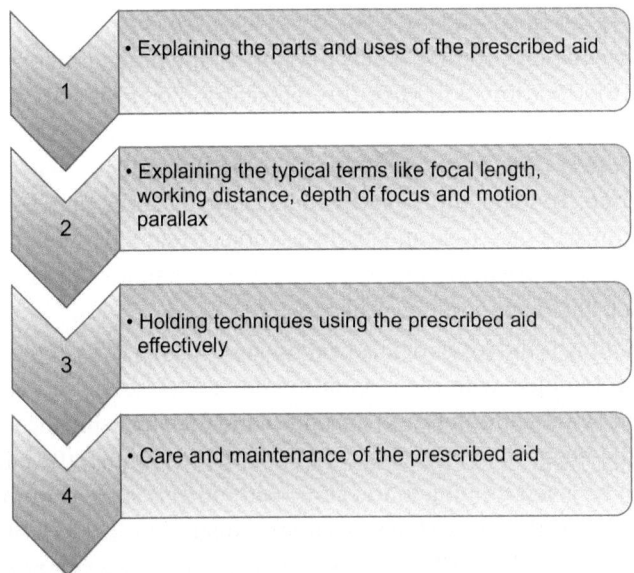

Flowchart 14.2: Sequential process for distance viewing training.

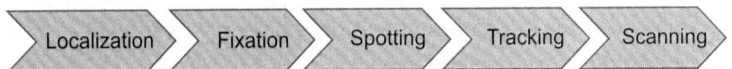

Localization training is teaching the patient to align the aid with the eye's line of sight using telescope. Training starts in the clinical practice with a few simple visual stimuli. The practitioner should stand in front of a blank front and focus the telescope at 10 feet distance. Then he should walk down to a position that is 10 feet in front of the patient and ask him to locate him. The patient with central scotoma must learn how to view eccentrically without aid before using the aid. Patient with multiple scotoma will find an object appears, disappears, and reappears in the field of view as its image passes through the several scotomas on retina. Sometimes it may be helpful to patch the eye except for a small opening in the patch that is placed where the practitioner thinks the best line of sight. The procedure helps the ocular muscles to develop a sense of directionalization to the visual stimuli and in time the patient develops localization skills.

Once the localization skill is developed, the practitioner should teach the fixation skill with the telescope. Fixation skill allows the patient to identify the object whose position is found through localization. This is achieved by teaching the patient focusing of telescope. To focus on a nearby object, the distance between the lenses must be increased and for distant object it should be decreased. Initially, the patient should focus slowly and practice blurring and clearing the image as often as necessary.

Spotting is the result of localization and fixation skills. It involves finding an object with the aid, raising the aid telescope so that it is aligned between the eyes and the object and then focusing the object until the image is as clear as possible. At the beginning, the patient should be given training in the clinic with objects such as numbers and letters on the walls which are larger enough to be located without the aid. As the skill builds up, the size of the object can be reduced and the distance can be increased and illumination level can also be varied. When the skill is mastered in sitting position, the activities can be repeated while the patient is standing. This is very important skill to use bioptic telescope effectively.

Then the patient is given training on tracking moving object. Tracking is the ability to follow a moving object in the environment. In order to track an object, the patient has to move his head at a speed determined by the speed of the movement of the object. Sometimes head movement has to be coupled with body movement. Eye movement is not allowed while tracking an object. Patient with central scotoma and peripheral scotoma will always find difficulties in tracking moving objects. Since tracking requires patients to move their head which is normally discouraged in the orientation and mobility training program, such patients usually get confused. It is, therefore, important that a collaborative training program is designed for such patients with the orientation and mobility instructor to avoid confusions.

Once the patient is able to track with telescope, last in line is scanning which is the most difficult but most valuable skill to enhance the maximum visual efficiency. Scanning is searching an object in the visual environment with the telescope. An effective visual scanning should follow a pattern, starting from an environmental reference point and ending at another environmental reference point while looking for an object on a cluttered wall to determine the length of the swaths. In the absence of any environmental reference, the patient must learn to use kinesthetic awareness to determine the swaths. Patients who are poor in using kinesthetic awareness should be encouraged to use the movement of their torso as they would be able to judge the length of the swaths by the amount of tension created in their torso.

Most patients are prescribed telescopes for distance and intermediate viewing tasks. Broadly, telescopes are two types—handheld monocular telescopes and spectacle mounted binocular telescopes. Handheld telescope is normally used when refractive correction in place, if the patient needs. The use of handheld telescope is relatively easier. The patient is instructed to spot the target without the telescope and then use telescope for focusing. However, binocular telescope mounted in spectacle is relatively difficult. The position of eyepiece is adjusted with patient's pupillary distance and the patient is instructed to adopt the head position that aligns the eyes with telescopic lenses, usually it happens with lowering the chin and then he is asked to read the test chart and then look around the room. Focusable binocular telescope should be adjusted for focus using both hands. Alignment to targets may be verified simply by asking the patient whether the image is circular. If bioptic telescope is used, the patient must first locate the target using carrier lenses and then he should drop his head down to bring the target into view with the telescope.

TRAINING FOR NEAR VIEWING AIDS

Near vision tasks include those activities with the need for visual acuity to perform tasks within 20 inches. These include common tasks such as:

- Reading
- Writing
- Crafts
- Sewing

The common low vision devices that will aid a patient in performing these tasks are shown in **Flowchart 14.3**.

The first step while providing training to a low vision patient is to identify the blind areas or scotomas. The patient with central scotomas or central visual field loss are highly benefitted by eccentric viewing. Eccentric viewing is an effective way for individuals with central scotomas to improve the use of the vision that they have. The literature shows that eccentric viewing training can improve near visual acuity and reading speed in people with central visual field loss. Once eccentric viewing has been discussed, the practitioner can move on to providing training on the proper use of device and its use for achieving reading goals.

Though a near vision aid is provided to perform some reading task, not all reading tasks are similar as they may require the need for different aid and different set of training instructions. For example, reading hotel menu card is different from reading newspaper or signing cheques. In addition to optical near viewing aid, the patient may also be prescribed nonoptical aid. Nonoptical aids may be used together with the optical aid and otherwise also.

After the patient develops the basic familiarities with eccentric viewing technique, the examiner should address following issues:
- Establishing and maintaining the correct focal distance of the prescribed aid
- Keeping one's place while reading
- Head and eye movement

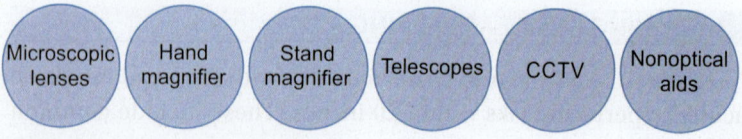

Flowchart 14.3: Common aids for near vision tasks.

(CCTV: closed-circuit television)

Microscopic Lenses

To establish the correct focal distance with microscopic lenses, the patient is trained to bring the reading material to his nose and then to push it back until a clear focus is obtained. Patient is told not to move the head and eye, instead scroll the reading material in front of them, similar to the typewriter's carriage. If the patient moves his head and eye, the focal distance will change, resulting in blur vision or distorted vision.

Handheld Magnifier

To establish the correct focal distance with handheld magnifier, the magnifier is laid on the page and then lifted until the best focus is attained. The page can be scrolled beneath the magnifier as the patient maintains the best eccentric viewing position. The hand magnifier is held parallel to the reading material so that the line of sight can be perpendicular to the lens. To minimize the peripheral distortion, the most curved side (Cx side) of the magnifier lens is held toward the patient's eyes.

Stand Magnifier

The patient is not required to hold the stand magnifier, instead it is supported by its housing that rests on the reading material. There are two types of stand magnifier:
1. Fixed focus stand magnifier
2. Focusable stand magnifier

In order to use the stand magnifier, put the reading material either on the flat surface of the table or on inclined stand or improvise with a clip board propped up on the book. Adjust the light to shine on the material at an angle to avoid reflection from the surface. Keep the stand magnifier pushing against the page while reading, and never lift it. If plano convex stand is used, a dark strip of paper is taped across the bottom of the lens to help isolate the line being read. Focusable stand magnifier is designed to be used with the eyes close to the lens. Typoscopes may be used to place over the reading material to increase contrast or block glare from surrounding page.

Reading Telescope

While providing training for handheld monocular telescope, the first step is to train the patient as to holding the telescope and practice rotating the eyepiece and then show the patient how to raise the monocular telescope to eye level and focus on reading material. Those patients who are prescribed telescope for distance viewing task may use the same for reading by placing a reading cap on the objective lens. Adding a reading cap of different power creates a different working distance and enables the patient to manage reading with the same telescopic lens.

Closed-Circuit Television

Closed-circuit television (CCTV) is a very useful tool when copious amount of reading and writing is to be done and also when the patient is not responding to optical aid because of the need for higher magnification, contrast, or problem with eccentric viewing technique. There are three major components of CCTV—camera, monitor, and movable reading platform. The patient needs to be trained on adjusting the height of the monitor so that viewing can be comfortable at the eye-level height. Another set of instructions are critical for placing the reading material on movable platform which is designed to be positioned underneath the camera. The majority of CCTV systems is accompanied by a built-in illumination source. Reflected glare can be controlled with the adjustments of manual controls for brightness, contrast, color, and image polarity. Glare effect can also be minimized by tilting the monitor, adjusting room lights, or placing the monitor in a location in which natural and artificial light does not reflect off the equipment surface.

Loss of peripheral fields can further complicate the prescription and subsequent training programs as it inhibits the information processing abilities of the visual system because not enough information is taken in at one time. To compensate for this deficiency, the patient must be trained to systematically scan the environment to obtain meaningful information. A thorough knowledge of size, location, and extent of field loss is critical before initiating the prescription of any aid and subsequent training program.

Chapter 14: Patient's Training

SELECT THE CORRECT ANSWER

1. Which of the following explains the main objective patient training in low vision care?
   a. To help low vision patient use his residual vision more effectively either with low vision aids or without low vision aids
   b. To help low vision patient use his residual vision more effectively with low vision aids
   c. To help low vision patient use his residual vision more effectively without low vision aids
   d. To make the low vision patient functionally independent

2. Which of the following is the main objective of training a low vision patient for developing localization skill while using telescopes?
   a. Patient develops the ability to follow a moving object with telescope
   b. Patient develops the ability of searching objects in the visual environment with telescope
   c. Patient develops a sense of directionalization to the visual stimulus
   d. Patient develops the ability to align the eyes with the object

3. Which of the following is not relevant while imparting training to a low vision patient for developing tracking ability to follow a moving object?
   a. Moving head is mandatory while tracking a moving object
   b. Eye movement is must be done
   c. Head movement has to be coupled with body movement
   d. Tracking is the ability to follow a moving object

4. Which of the following condition suggests that the patient must learn the art of eccentric viewing technique first before using the low vision aids efficiently?
   a. Patient with ring scotoma
   b. Patient with multiple scotoma
   c. Patient with relative scotoma
   d. Patient with central scotoma

5. Which of the following is effective approach to minimize the effect of glare while reading?
   a. Use of nonoptical aid
   b. Correct positioning of light source
   c. Adjustment of room lights
   d. All of the above

Answers

| 1. a | 2. c | 3. b | 4. d | 5. d |

SELF-PRACTICING QUESTIONS

1. Write a detailed note on training eccentric viewing technique to a low vision patient with central visual field loss.
2. Write an illustrative note differentiating between how would you like to provide training to a low vision patient for using distance low vision aid and near low vision aids.

15 CHAPTER

Orientation and Mobility Training

Chapter Outline
- Functional Orientation and Mobility Evaluation
- Mobility Aids and Technique

The complete vision rehabilitation program needs engagement of various disciplines because the patient may have different visual goals and their visual performance may vary depending on visual conditions and environmental circumstances. Orientation and mobility training **(Fig. 15.1)** services are one of the important areas of overall rehabilitation training program which is used to help patient

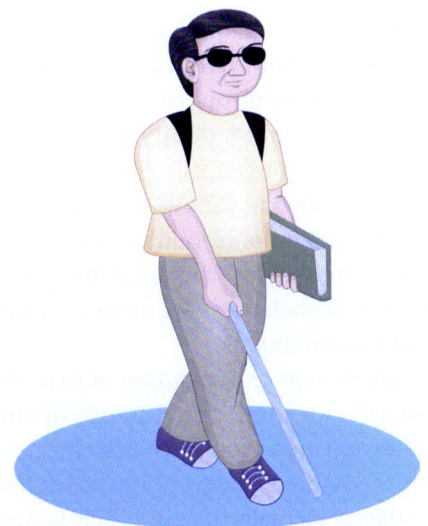

Fig. 15.1: Walking stick training

with low vision maintain travel independence. Orientation stands for awareness of position in space and mobility implies the capability of moving about through the environment safely, efficiently, and independently. All low vision patients may not need orientation and mobility training, but those who are unable to move about with ease and independently may be gradually exposed to the situations such as traveling in residential, school, or business areas and using public transportation. Successful mobility depends on the effective use of visual information rather than visual acuity. The other variables which affect mobility training are peripheral field defects, light levels, and contrast sensitivity. Some patients can be made self-sufficient with the use of low vision travel devices. For others whose problems are not completely solved with these devices, the referral for an orientation and mobility evaluation is indicated. The mobility instructor performs a functional vision assessment to evaluate mobility potential and plan a training program emphasizing effective use of vision and other senses. Recommended travel aids are incorporated into the program.

FUNCTIONAL ORIENTATION AND MOBILITY EVALUATION

Before starting a training program, the visually impaired patients should have a thorough low vision evaluation and with due considerations obtained from the case history, the functional evaluation for orientation and mobility program is started. This evaluation has to be done at night as well as during the day. If the patient needs to be evaluated in various areas such as residential, a college campus, business, indoors, outdoors, or any other specific surrounding-evaluation may be scheduled for several sessions to avoid over fatigue. Certain behaviors are observed in all settings and under different lighting conditions.

- *Distances for identifying and avoiding objects*: The instructor notes the size, color, texture, and distance of objects that the patient identifies and then avoids. Whether he identifies moving objects or only the stationary objects are also noted. Whether he identifies the objects tactually or auditorially before using vision is also noted.

- *Determination of movement*: Detection of direction and distance of traffic, pedestrians, and others are also noted.
- *Scanning pattern*: Whether the patient scans more to one side than the other is also noted.
- *Fixation*: Whether the patient looks directly at the object or the side or slightly up or down. Whether staring at an object causes nystagmus or not?
- *Landmarks used for orientation*: The examiner would like to know what clues and landmarks, does the patient use for orientation? If the patient uses visual landmark, do they have a common characteristic such as same size, color, relative location, and so forth.
- *Use of color*: Does the patient identify a particular color more easily than other? How does the lighting affect the ability to identify and use color?

MOBILITY AIDS AND TECHNIQUE

Although there are many mobility aids, five types of visual aids are used for mobility:
1. Conventional glasses or contact lenses
2. Glare and illumination controlling aids such as absorptive lenses
3. Magnification aids such as handheld monocular telescope and head-borne bioptic telescopes
4. Minifying devices
5. Prisms and mirrors that relocate image

Some low vision patients may need to use nonvisual techniques to supplement vision under unfavorable conditions such as night, unfamiliar territory, or inclement weather. Six types of nonvisual aids are either used alone or in combination with visual aids:
1. Sighted guide, i.e., holding arm of sighted person
2. Long cane or support cane
3. Protective arm technique to avoid contact or injury to upper and lower body
4. Trailing, i.e., following a wall with the back of hand
5. Dog guide
6. Electronic aids.

Chapter 15: Orientation and Mobility Training

SELECT THE CORRECT ANSWER

1. What does orientation mean in reference to training a patient with low vision?
   a. Knowing where you are and where you want to go
   b. A meeting at the beginning of the session
   c. The ability to move around safely
   d. A spot where you want the patient to fixate at

2. Which of the following variable does not affect mobility training for a low vision patient?
   a. Peripheral field defects
   b. Light levels
   c. Ability of patient to process visual information
   d. Ability of patient's bodily muscle to stretch

3. Which of the following is not considered as mobility skill?
   a. Ability to walk without tripping or falling
   b. Ability to locate oneself in one's environment
   c. Ability to cross streets
   d. Use of public transportation

Answers

| 1. a | 2. d | 3. b |

SELF-PRACTICING QUESTION

1. Write down your opinion on how can translating information into auditory message help low vision patient during orientation and mobility training.

16 CHAPTER

Low Vision Practice Management

Chapter Outline
- Setting Up the Low Vision Clinic
- Setting Up the Fees Structure
- Referrals
- Letter Writing
- Practice Model
- Patient Recall

There is quite a bit of difference in common vision care practice and low vision practice. In common practice, people come to the optometrists when they find some difficulties in seeing objects either at far or at near and extended near distance or with symptoms. The optometrist tests their eyes on high contrast Snellen chart in an environment of ideal room light, static position, and high visual stimulus and prescribes them a correction that enables them to read 20/20 or 6/6 line clearly. Or, he examines the patient in slit lamp, diagnose, try to locate the signs relevant to their symptoms and refer them to an ophthalmologist for appropriate treatment. In common practice, patients are the passive recipient of care, whereas optometrists are the dominant professional—one giving expert advice or suggestions or consultations and other carrying them out. The practice of low vision is completely different.

Almost all patients have poor vision. Moreover, they have been told on several occasions that nothing can be done to improve their visual condition and they have to live with their condition. The patients feel abandoned and psychologically experience a big let-down. When they get the opportunity to visit a low vision practitioner as because someone has referred them or they came to know through their sources, they carry huge expectations. This is the reason why the most part of initial interaction between patients and the practitioners is spent in removing the doubts from the patient's mind, build up sensible expectations, and to encourage the patient to come out of hopelessness to regain the independence and self-respect.

Unlike the general eye examination, low vision examiner does not diagnose any eye disease or treat any ocular condition, instead he deals with already diagnosed ocular condition and look at the possibility of using the residual visual acuity to restore the functional independence of the patient. The low vision practitioner starts from a point where the ophthalmologists have denied any further help, considers the patient's visual condition, his psychological status, the effect socioeconomic factors and available types of low vision aids, and finally shows them a new way to be functionally independent.

There are multiple services for the complete low vision rehabilitation program. No single profession can provide all the services; the ophthalmologist, the optometrist, the orientation and mobility instructor, the counselor, the educator all add parts to the whole from which the patient must select what is most helpful. Low vision patients are taught to use their remaining visual abilities, much like physical or occupational therapists would help an individual who has suffered from a stroke. By adapting appliances and utilizing vision rehabilitation devices specially designed for the needs of the individual, many individuals with low vision are able to maintain their functional independence.

Low vision is completely a specialized area of optometry that needs specialized training. The complete low vision examination takes time and is usually completed in more than one session. In fact, low vision rehabilitation is the beginning of services that has to be continued throughout the life. Apart from examination, training is also the important element of low vision practice. Patient's engagement is very critical. In fact, a demonstration of the different types of aids is the key. Patients are demonstrated the effectivity of different aids and they are explained how the use of those aids will help them become functionally independent. It is, therefore, a collaborative effort of patient and the practitioner. Besides the patient's readiness to accept the limitations is also very important. The low vision specialist shows the way and the patient needs to follow him.

Although the scope seems to be quite a big, the science could not gain the desired acceptance because of lot of barriers:
- Limited awareness
- Lack of professional referral system
- Lack of resource materials
- Not many institutions provide education on low vision services
- Lack of standardization in service
- Primary focus on selling aids with very limited follow-ups.
- No fixed recognized certification program
- Advanced tools are very expensive and are not easily available.

In practice, it has been noticed that most low vision patients visit the low vision clinic very late. Early intervention is critical for children and young patients with visual impairments as it builds a foundation for further learning. They may be encouraged to use not only their residual vision but also other senses to make sense of their world. Even for elderly patients' intervention at the early stage of the disease increases the effectivity of the low vision devices. It has been recognized world over, but the lack of awareness and lack of professional referral system hinders the practical implications of these programs. The adaptation to visual impairment reduces dependency on others and enhances the functional dependence. When this is combined with the passion to prove one's own ability, there is a possibility of great social recognition. Profound vision loss in adolescents, young adults, and middle-aged adults is associated with significant negative psychological and psychosocial effects, which are influenced by age and social surroundings. Aging adds further difficulties. Tremors, inability to grasp the instructions for focusing the aid and position it correctly, poor hand and eye coordination, reduced auditory system, and over expectations are really frustrating. The purpose of intervention with low vision patient is not only remedial but also include development of intentional functioning.

SETTING UP THE LOW VISION CLINIC

A low vision clinic can be started from the very simplest level by including considerations of prescribing simplest magnifier right up to the full grown low vision practice. A full grown low vision practice should have all the tests needed to conduct an effective low vision examination and also all types of low vision aids. The following set of equipment needed to set up an effective low vision aid clinic:

- High and low LogMAR charts
- Snellen test chart
- Near vision test charts
- Retinoscope
- Amsler grid test
- Tangent screen
- Full aperture trial lens set
- Ishihara test chart
- Farnsworth Munsell D15 test
- Contrast sensitivity test
- Glare test
- Reading stand
- Lux meter
- Clip board
- A set of microscopic glasses
- A set of magnifier
- A set of telescope for distance vision
- A set of telescope for near vision
- A set of nonoptical aids
- A set of absorptive lenses
- Pinhole spectacle
- Pinhole contact lenses
- A set of field expander aids
- Rheostat room light

SETTING UP THE FEES STRUCTURE

Low vision practice is a specialized area of optometry and it should not be undervalued. Therefore, revenue model needs to be established at the outset. There are different models of practice and fees structure has to be designed based upon the model of practice. If you set up your own clinic, you may charge professional fees based upon number of hours of engagement during per visit. The fees for first consultation may be little more than the follow-up consultation. An additional fee may be charged for training of low vision aids. Appliances such as magnifiers, telescopes, microscopic lenses, contact lenses, or any other are invoiced separately. Retainer ship fee model may be implemented depending upon the credentials of your acquaintances. The only disadvantage of this model of practice is that you might have to be available at any time at a moment's notice.

REFERRALS

There is a very famous old phrase that says, "What you're doing speaks so loudly that I cannot hear what you're saying." This is very important for getting referrals and when it comes to low vision practice, referrals are the Holy Grail. Ophthalmologists and eye hospitals where the patients are diagnosed and treated for eye diseases are the biggest sources of referrals. Satisfied and happy patients can be the brand ambassador of the practice. Special education schools can be one of the biggest sources of referrals. But getting referrals from them are not easier. You must establish your credibility as a low vision expert. Credibility is the feeling of trust and respect that you inspire in others for yourself. It is not easy to establish credibility because no single thing creates credibility. A host of things should be in place for on and on. Integrity, commitment, and honesty are three building blocks for establishing the credibility. In professional practice, integrity is all about providing great solutions to the patients that makes difference in their lives. Commitment refers to personal dedication and aspirations to excel and master what you do and honesty implies that you care for your patient genuinely. You need to shape what they think about you and it has to be insanely patient caring and memorable in their minds as unique to you. When you develop such credibility, you become linked as default recommendations for your specialized service.

Rehabilitation is like a big umbrella and there are several professional services under it. Low vision practitioner may often need to work with professionals like orientation and mobility instructor, the counselor, the educator, all add parts to the whole from which the patient can be benefitted. Low vision practitioner may develop his own network with them that can enable him to create a chain of patients. The best referrals come about patient has had an opportunity to experience the value that you are capable of delivering.

In this epic era of digital world leveraging social media may help you create multiple avenues for referrals. You just need to deliver news by way of writing articles and blogs about how your practice has helped patients in different ways. A constant flow of news circulation in the form of story helps a lot to spread your credibility.

However, managing referrals are critical to gain referrals constantly. Your advocates expect acknowledgement. These acknowledgements may be in different forms depending upon your relationship with them. But personalized hand written simple letter always works very effectively in most cases. Some practices send gift vouchers together with letters, while others send gifts in kind. You need to be very time sensitive for gaining regular referrals from your advocates. Unless the referral management is well-coordinated, it can be very frustrating or even dangerous.

LETTER WRITING

Letter writing is one of the important element of low vision practice. Low vision practitioner may often write letters to school teachers regarding capabilities of the student, need for the use of low vision devices, instructional tips in using the devices, and suggestions for preferential seating, etc. It may also be needed to convey information to the doctors and counselors. Whenever a referral from an ophthalmologist is received, a short report on evaluation and performance of the patient is also important. Letter writing may take lot of time. It is, therefore, always recommended to have fixed formats ready for different types of letters.

Chapter 16: Low Vision Practice Management

PRACTICE MODEL

The low vision model is different from general eye examination practice model because of the following reasons:
- A typical low examination takes more time than what is needed for general eye examination. It may be split in three sessions as shown in **Flowchart 16.1**. These sessions may be on different dates or as mutually convenient. Though many practitioners are of opinion that the patients hoping to obtain some help, they must be given enough time in the initial visit only to maintain their enthusiasm. But it does not work consistently in the long run. The possible reasons may be enumerated as under:
  - Patient may be tired which may affect his engagement.
  - Most patients do not come with the intention of buying aid in the first visit.
  - It is against the commercial interest of the practice. If the practice does not yield sufficient commercial benefits from the practice as compared to time invested, it cannot survive for long.

  It is, therefore, prudent to keep the first session for examination and counseling, second session may be totally dedicated to the demonstration of different types of low vision aids and when the prescription for aids is finalized, the practitioner may call the patient for training of the application of prescribed aids.
- Most patients in low vision practice are either children or old. It is always difficult to rush with them as they take time to understand and get into the desirable state of mind for the positive outcomes of the evaluation. However, the practitioner may have flexible approach with those patients who respond quickly and engage themselves with the practitioner to get benefits out of the practice.

Flowchart 16.1: Objective of different sessions.

First session	• Evaluation and counseling
Second session	• Demonstration of aids
Final session	• Training of aids

The objective of the practice is never to follow the rules rigidly but to deliver the effective services so that patient gets his objective met and the practitioner also gets his due rewards.
- There are many practitioners who advocate the loaning system for aids but the author is totally against such practice as it is in most cases detrimental to the practice and also it affects patient's effort to embrace the aid. Either their effort is constantly in search of looking for further scope of improvement or they look for alternative sources for buying aids. Both are not good for practice and patient in any manner.

PATIENT RECALL

Recall of patients is essential to monitor the visual status and ocular health of the patient, as well as to monitor the effectiveness of the prescribed devices. Also, the practitioner may be interested to talk to the patient regarding new developments.

To sum up low vision practice has tremendous potential to deliver. Ophthalmologists need to understand that they refer the patient to low vision specialist as soon as possible so that patient gets full benefits and the science is also recognized. The science is growing across the world and sophisticated aids are manufactured. Time is not far when there will be several aid manufacturers who will come forward to make their effort to develop the science same as contact lens manufacturer are making efforts to develop contact lens market.

SELF-PRACTICING QUESTION

1. What are the minimum set of test tools and low vision devices would you like to recommend to set up a low vision clinic in private practice?

Bibliography

1. Benjamin WJ. (ed). Borish's Clinical Refraction. Oxford: Butterworth-Heinemann; 2006.
2. Bier N. Correction of Subnormal Vision. London: Butterworth & Co Publishers Ltd; 1970.
3. Brilliant R, Graboyes M. Set Realistic Goals for Low-Vision Care: Pay attention to the whole person, not just the vision loss, and find out what the patient wants to achieve. [online] Available from: https://www.reviewofoptometry.com/article/set-realistic-goals-for-low-vision-care. [Last accessed January 2022].
4. Brilliant RL. Essentials of Low Vision Practice. Oxford: Butterworth-Heinemann; 1998.
5. Dagnelie G. Age-related psychophysical changes and low vision. Invest Ophthalmol Vis Sci. 2013;54(14):ORSF88-93.
6. Duke Elder S, Abrams D, (eds). System of Ophthalmology. London: Kimpton; 1971.
7. Faye EE. (ed). Clinical Low Vision. Philadelphia: Lippincott Williams and Wilkins; 1984.
8. Hyon JY, Yeo HE, Seo JM, Lee IB, Lee JH, Hwang JM. Objective measurement of distance visual acuity determined by computerized optokinetic nystagmus test. Invest Ophthalmol Vis Sci. 2010;51(2):752-7.
9. Jose RT. (ed). Understanding Low Vision. Arlington County: American Foundation for the Blind; 1983.
10. Know about Different Types of Lights in Lighting System, By Dave, July 22, 2019.
11. Lowth M. (2016). Visual Field Defects. [online] Available from: scribd.com/document/347244695/Visual-Field-Defects. [Last accessed January 2022].
12. Melore GG, London R. (eds). Treating Vision Problems in the Older Adult. Missouri: Mosby Inc.; 1997.
13. Meriano C, Latella D. Occupational Therapy Interventions: Function and Occupation. West Deptford: Slack Incorporated; 2016.
14. Punani B, Rawal N. Visual Impairment Handbook. New Delhi: Ashish Publishing House; 1993.
15. Rosenthal BP, Cole RG, (eds). Functional Assessment of Low Vision. Netherlands: Elsevier; 1995.

Bibliography

WEBSITE REFERENCES

- www.emedicene.com
- www.ocutech.com
- www.athenaeye.com
- www.eyeassociates.com
- www.thomson-software-solutions.com
- www.visionrx.com
- www.tsbvi.edu
- www.banjoben.com
- www.spedex.com
- www.rnib.org.uk
- www.vard.org
- www.achromat.org
- www.theretinasource.com
- www.maculardegeneration.org
- www.socco.edu
- www.sbsystems_design.com
- www.vhct.org
- www.vision.psych.umn.edu
- www.caramity.org.uk
- www.albinism.org
- www.slsbvi.org
- www.eschenbach.com
- www.contrastsensitivity.net
- www.city.ac.uk

Index

Page numbers followed by *f* refer to figure, *fc* refer to flowchart and *t* refer to table.

A

Absorptive lenses 139, 140*f*, 166
    set of 190
Achromatopsia 87
Advanced low vision aids 146
Age-related macular degeneration 26, 77, 88, 104
Albinism 91, 92*f*
    contact lens for 145
Amblyopia 5
Amsler chart with lines 72*f*
Amsler grid
    chart 69, 74*f*
    test 68, 74*t*, 190
Angular magnification 110
Aniridia 96
    contact lens for 145
Antireflection coating 141
Autorefractometer 44

B

Bailey and Lovie charts 28
Bar magnifier 127, 127*f*
Bifocal microscopes 123
Big shot screen magnifier 156, 157*f*
Binocular aid 164
Binocular visual field 67*f*
Bioptic telescope 132, 133*f*
Bioptic telescopic spectacle 168
Black felt tip pen 135
Blind spots 88
Blurred vision 95, 98, 100, 104
Braille display systems 154
Braille translation software 154*f*

C

Caps 96, 136
Cataract 100
Central scotomas 26, 94
Central vision
    loss of 3, 4*f*
    management of 94
    progressive loss of 95
Central visual field
    defect 67
    loss 104
Chart design 29
Classic half-eye microscopes 122
Clip board 190
Closed-circuit television 74, 94, 103, 146, 147*f*, 163, 164, 178, 180
    system 111
Coloboma 99
Color defects 104

Color perception, loss of 1
Color vision 92
    contact lens for loss of 145
    loss of 90
    test 51, 52*f*
Color, use of 185
Complete vision rehabilitation program 183
Comprehensive low vision examination 14
Computer-assisted devices 150, 150*fc*
    assessment for 155
    development of 150
Cone malformation 88
Confrontation technique 76, 77*f*
Contact lens 51, 95, 144-146, 166
Contrast sensitivity 1, 79
    assessment, methods for 81
    test 79, 80, 190
        charts for 82
        need for 81
Cornea 102
Corneal opacity 5
Corning color protect filter 103
Corning photo chromatic filter 141
Crystalline lens 100
Current visual status 63

D

Daily living, activities of 20
Deficient color vision 94
Diabetes, juvenile 3
Diabetic retinopathy 5, 77, 90
    effect of 90*f*
Dim illumination 88, 96
Distance
    magnification 112
    viewing aids, training for 174
    vision 20, 190
    visual acuity, measuring 26

E

Effective low vision counselling, components of 62
Eyes, irregular rapid movement of 92

F

Factors affecting visual acuity test 24
Farnsworth-Munsell D-15 test 52, 52*f*, 190
Feinbloom charts 28, 28*f*
Field expansion
    channel lens 142, 169
    devices, three types of 142*fc*
Filters 88
    lenses 50
Fixation 185

Index

Fixed focus stand magnifier 179
    disadvantages of 126
Flexibility 58
Flexible test distance 41
Fluctuating vision 90
Fluorescent light 118
Focusable stand magnifier 179
Fresnel lens 128
Fresnel magnifier 127, 127*f*
Fresnel prism 142, 143*f*, 169
Full aperture trial lens set 190
Full field
    microscopes 122
    telescope 131
Functional acuity contrast test 84
    chart 84*f*

G

Galilean telescope 129, 167, 167*t*
    reverse 143
Ghost image 103
Glare 5, 20, 85, 101
    direct 85
    disability 84
    effect 104
    indirect 85
    problem 99
    test 79, 84, 190
Glass, single magic pair of 10
Glaucoma 3, 5, 77, 96, 97*f*
Grief, five stages of 6*fc*, 7

H

Half-eye microscopes 122
Half-eye microscopic lenses 123*f*
Halogen light 117
Handheld concave lens 144
Handheld magnifier 124, 179
    focal distance of 125*f*
Hardware-based low vision aids 151
Hazy vision 100*f*
Hemianopia 3, 77, 103
    altitudinal 67
    bitemporal 67
    homonymous 67, 103*f*, 170
Hemianopsia, bitemporal 171
High contrast Snellen chart 187
High Logmar charts 190
High myopes, contact lens for 144
High myopia 5
High refractive error 92
Histoplasmosis 77, 94

I

Illumination 115, 134
    distribution 118
    quality 118
    quantity 118
    sources of 117
Image compressing 143
Intraocular fungal infection 94
Intraocular infection, severe 91
Inwave field-expanding channel lens 143*f*
Iris 96
Ishihara chart 52*f*, 190

J

Jaws 156
    screen reader 156*f*

K

Keplerian telescope 130, 167, 167*t*
Keratoconus 102, 102*f*, 103
    contact lens for 145
Keratometer 44
Kestenbaum rule 36

L

Large aperture trial lenses 43
Large letter cards 134*f*
Lens
    clouding 100*f*
    large changes of 43
Letter chart determines 83
Light 5, 20
    adaptation, management of 94
    artificial 117
    emitting diode 117
    from object, reflection of 115
    incandescent 117
    natural 117
Lighthouse method 36, 37
Lighthouse near test
    card 34
    chart 32
Logmar chart 29, 30, 31*f*
    advantages of 32
Logmar units 30
Logmar value 30
Low contrast letter test 83
Low Logmar charts 190
Low vision 1, 2, 2*f*, 13, 19, 24, 68, 81, 87, 174, 188
    aids 88, 89, 91, 92, 94-99, 101, 103, 104, 121, 139, 144, 160
    software-based 152
    types of 121*fc*
    clinical characteristics of 3
    common causes of 87
    counseling 62*fc*
    examination 13, 16*fc*, 18
        objective of 40
    history taking 19*t*
    management 74

Index

practice 23, 190
  management 187
  principles of 9, 9*fc*
psychology of 6
refraction 39, 42*fc*, 49
stuff 7
visual symptoms of 104*t*
Lux meter 190

M

Macula 88, 94, 95
Macular degeneration 89*f*
Macular holes 77
Magic magnification software 156
Magnifications 107
  and lens power scheme 109*t*, 110*t*
  power of 111
Magnifier 123
  general principles of 124
  set of 190
  types of 124, 124*fc*
Microscopic glasses, set of 190
Microscopic lenses 122, 179
Mirrors 169
  system 104
MN read test chart 32, 33*f*
Mobile speak talking mobile phone software 158
Monocular telescopes 89
Monocular visual field 66*f*
Movement, determination of 185
Multiple field loss 104
Mydriasis, artificial 69

N

Near magnification 113
Near viewing aids 161
  training for 177
Near vision 20, 88, 174, 190
  acuity 36
    test 32
  tasks 177
    common aids for 178*fc*
  test charts 190
  types of aids for 162*fc*
Needle threader 138, 138*f*
Neodymium light 117
Night blindness 5, 94, 104
  management of 94
Night vision aid 138
Nonfocusable stand magnifier 126*f*
Nonoptical aids 133
  set of 190
Notex 138, 138*f*
Nystagmus 88, 92, 96, 97, 99, 100

O

Object, distance of 110
Objective 69
  method 44
  refraction, mechanics of 44*fc*
Ocular condition, impact of 63
Ocular diseases 77
Ocutech bioptic telescope 148*f*
Ocutech vision enhancing systems 148
Optic atrophy 77, 98
Optic nerve 96, 98
Optical aids 96, 122
  types of 122*fc*
Optotypes 29
Overall blurred vision 3, 5, 5*f*

P

Pelli-Robson chart 83*f*
Peripheral fields, loss of 180
Peripheral vision 95
  loss of 3, 4*f*, 94
Peripheral visual
  field defect 67, 170
  impairment 98
Photophobia 97, 99, 101, 165
  extreme 88, 96
  painful 92
Photostress 95
Pigments
  partial loss of 91
  total loss of 91
Pinhole 50
  contact lens 59, 96, 145*f*, 190
  spectacle 139, 139*f*, 166, 190
Poor central vision 88
Poor contrast 6*f*, 104
Prism 50
  lenses 104
Projection chart 35
Projection magnification 111

Q

Quick fix method 10

R

Random dots Amsler chart 72*f*
Reading
  stand 135, 136*f*, 190
  telescope 180
Recording visual acuity score 30, 35
Reflecting mirror 144
Refraction procedure 43, 44*f*
Refractive correction 59
Rehabilitation 192

Index

Retina 88, 90, 91, 93
    peripheral 94
    rods of 92
Retinal detachment 77, 101
Retinal illuminance 166, 168, 168t
Retinal pigmentary degeneration 92
Retinitis pigmentosa 3, 5, 77, 92, 93f
Retinoscope 190
Retinoscopy 45, 47
Rheostat room light 190
Rigid gas permeable 103, 166
Room illumination 25

S

Scotoma 67
    location of 74
Semi reflective planomirror 144f
Setting up low vision clinic 190
Sine-wave contrast test 82
    chart 82f
Sloan letters 29
Snellen chart 13, 27, 27f, 28, 190
Spectacle lens 139, 143f, 166
Spectacle magnifier 162
Speech recognition system 153
Squint, development of 100
Stand magnifier 125, 162, 179
Standard Amsler grid chart 70f, 71f
Stargardt diseases 95
Static visual acuity 165
Stenopaic slit 50
Strabismus 99
Sunglasses 88, 96

T

Table lamps 135f
Tactile products 137
Tactile telephone 137f
Talking products 137
Talking telephone 137f
Tangent screen 75, 75f, 190
    test 75
Telemicroscope 131, 132f
Telescope 59, 128, 128f, 129fc, 166, 168
    power of 132
    retinal illuminance of 168t
    set of 190
Telescopic lenses 111f
Telescopic system 146
Temporal field loss 144f
Test charts 24, 69
    placement of 42
Test distance 25, 29, 69
Total color blindness 87

Touch screen 152f
Toxoplasmosis 91
Traditional test charts 24
Tunnel vision 3, 96, 104
Typoscope 135, 136f

V

Vision 79
    loss 1
    peripheral field of 94
    reciprocal of 36, 37
    rehabilitation 89, 94
Visors 88, 96, 136
    use of 59
Visual acuity 1, 23, 25, 35, 88, 96, 99, 99f
    dynamic 165
    test 23, 24fc, 26t
    effect on 26
Visual behavior 14, 15, 15t
Visual comfort, improving 116
Visual concerns 20
Visual defects 88, 90, 91, 93, 94, 95, 96, 98, 100, 101, 102, 103
Visual field 26, 66, 88, 92, 99f, 100
    approximation of 77f
    constriction of 96
    defects 1, 67, 77t
        prescribing aids for 169
        tests for 68
        types of 67
    examination 66
    expanding aids 141
    loss 24, 26t, 90, 99, 101
    traits of 26
    test 66, 68f, 76
        objective of 66
        purpose of 68
Visual impairment, adaptive strategies for 24t
Visual rehabilitation 91
Visual task 116
Vocational and educational history 19

W

Walking stick training 183f

X

X-chrome contact lenses 146f, 166

Y

Younger protective lens series 141

Z

Zoom text xtra 157